Running Shoes
Are a Girl's Best Friend

Margreet Dietz

Copyright © 2009 by Margreet Dietz

First edition

All worldwide rights reserved. No part of this publication may be reproduced, stored in a retrieval system, or transmitted in any form or by any means, electronic, mechanical, photocopying, recording, or otherwise, without the prior written permission of the copyright owner of this book.

www.margreetdietz.com

Cover image: © Rezie Dietz-Wiesner

ISBN 978-1-4499583-9-8.

CONTENTS

Acknowledgements
Introduction 1
1. Pat Carroll: That sense of accomplishment is available to anyone   5
"It is really important to enjoy the journey rather than feel like it is something you have to do."

2. Susan Griffith: Exercise is a critical element to our wellbeing   13
"People who take running up later in life find that it gives them a level of confidence they didn't know existed."

3. Angela Adamson: It makes me happy   21
"I have 3 small children, work 4 days a week, and can honestly say that running is my release."

4. Anne-Maree Jaggs: Taking care of yourself is not selfish   24
"Cool wind in my hair on a hot afternoon, boosts of unexpected energy, and positive, unsolicited comments from people I least expect"

5. Running my first marathon was incredible (anonymous)   27
"You end up with some hyperventilating guy slapping around behind you and you slow down so you don't have to call an ambulance."

6. Becky Pratten: Motherhood provided the inspiration   33
"Running means freedom, self-expression and an identity other than being a mum."

7. Cassie Smith: Find the courage to try   37
"I give every training run the respect it deserves and try my hardest."

8. Christina Siu: Always give life a go   43
"Running has also taught me never to say never, and that doing something difficult and facing the challenge is so rewarding."

9. Davina Alston: Boost your confidence   46
"I love the atmosphere of the events that I compete in; I think the competitive air is really motivating and inspirational."

10. Diane Soffe: Taking charge of your destiny   51
"I realised there were two options left to me; I could continue to get old or I could do something about it."

11. Fiona Paul: It is my passion   58
"A great run feels like the hard work is getting easier."

12. Fiona Skinner: Forging lifelong bonds along the trails   66
"Running has brought me lots of good adventures, challenges and new friendships."

13. Gina Unwin: Determined to run again when told I wouldn't   69
"I feel very free when I run and lots of new ideas come to me."

14. Helen Bruce: It was easier than we thought   74
"It is all about getting into a routine that you can maintain for the rest of your life."

15. Helen: Running is my choice – and my success   80
"I used to run at 4:30am so no one would see me as I chased my dream."

16. Karen Scott: I didn't consider myself to be sporty   85
"The intensity and sacrifices involved in training for a marathon are all worthwhile when you realise, in the last 3km, that you are about to complete the biggest challenge of your life so far."

17. Karey Corrie: Effort brings surprising results   92
"Running gives me confidence to be true to myself and reminds me to push my own limits regularly, both on the road and in life in general."

18. Katrina Crook: Looking for an age group I can win   97
"Races gave me the motivation to keep running. I kept every certificate, timing list and T-shirt from the first few years."

19. Keryn Clark: Take control of your destiny   104
"For all its connotations with discipline and routine, it is a very user-friendly and flexible sport requiring minimum props and expense."

20. Lisa Hurring: A desire to run drove my rehabilitation   109
"It's a source of satisfaction and personal achievement that's always with me, no matter how other aspects of my life might be faring."

21. Elizabeth Bennett: Thoughts of a serial marathoner   116
"Running fits in as a matter of routine and as an unquestioned part of every day life."

22. Margot McGinness: My time is sacred   120
"I have completed eight half marathons, two marathons and countless shorter events - I still struggle to call myself a runner."

23. Shelley Kirkwood: Keeping my mind in check   124
"Any form of exercise has to be a lifestyle. It has to be woven into everyday life so that it becomes one of the things you just do."

24. Shelley Maxwell-Smith: The big hill I climbed   129
"I wanted to be one of those fit-looking girls."

25. Stacey Harland and Karen Bradley: The power of friendship   137
"When the alarm goes off I just have to get up and go whether I'm in a good or a bad mood because I know Stacey's waiting."

26. Stacia Nelson: From reluctance to commitment   142
"My partner used to ask me, 'When was your last run?' if I was a bit irritable. Too funny, he was usually right. I just need to go for a run."

27. Susan Trodd: Coping with menopause   147
"At 54, I decided that I was not going to let preconceptions of age stop me and to return to the interests of my youth - one being running."

28. Vicky Baxter-Wright: When my walking buddies didn't show   150
"A good run can also just be about the conversation we have as we run. Sometimes I've had to stop because I was laughing so much."

29. Victoria: Positively energised   154
"They think I'm obsessed with this running drug. That I do too much, it influences my social life too much and takes too much time away from them."

30. Virginia O'Connor: Pulling on my running shoes   159
"I had decided I wanted to run until I was at least six months pregnant but my body had other ideas and I chose to listen to it."

31. Aimee Barrett: The habit that I need to feel positive   163
"I feel it's what the human body has been designed for."

32. Anne Marie Halton: A great run makes me feel invincible   165
"I have more energy, am more motivated to take risks, I feel like I can do whatever I set my sights on given the right preparation."

33. Anne Jones: My life feels poorer without it   168
"Nothing quite equals the good feelings and the lift to my spirit that I get from running."

34. Caroline: Planning to ensure my training fits   172
"The realisation that slower runners are still real runners is one of my best experiences involving running."

35. Cathy Sheaff: Great legs are a good enough reason   176
"I haven't worked out what makes it a good run - if I did I'd plan to only have good runs."

36. Chris Jones: A long-time walker picks up her pace   178
"Running is to me proof that I have willpower - inner strength."

37. Colette Woodliffe: One too many glasses of champagne   181
"Running is supreme as it is freedom for body, mind and soul."

38. Deborah Kemp: The confidence will surprise you   184
"I ran 18km and I just could not believe it. I knew then that I could do a half marathon and it felt great to realise I had reached a new level."

39. Eileen Varty: Taking on more challenges   187
"I had a Birmingham hip replacement and went through a stage of maybe never running again which was totally devastating."

40. Elizabeth Adams: A marathon wasn't my objective   190
"Many people are amazed when you say have run a marathon."

41. Jan Roberts: My brother said I wouldn't last   192
"I am 48 and in very good shape. My mom says I have the body of a 25-year old. I say, 'Mom, I work really hard at it'."

42. Laura How: Freedom for my spirit   195
"I not only think about the health benefits, I also feel them as my body changes and I become stronger."

43. Manda Milling: A training program helps me focus   199
"My husband says I'm much nicer after I have been running."

44. Margo McLay: I realised that I like to compete   202
"I like the feeling of satisfaction that I get when I complete a significant race such as a 10km or a half marathon."

45. Rhonda LeBrocque: The healthier my body the better my life   204
"People think it is too hard but until you start you don't realise that it isn't that difficult at all and you don't have to be fast to be a runner."

46. Ros Holcombe: Being fit, looking good and staying young   207
"He encouraged me to try the China Coast half marathon. I thought he was nuts. But I did it."

47. Shannon Daley: A priority because I make it one   209
"Sometimes I will feel exhausted before a run but when I get back I am completely energised."

48. Sharon Varley: My pace sustains my love for the sport   212
"I love how I feel as a result of running - mentally and physically. It's a real outlet for me. It helps me keep a positive perspective on life"

49. Stephanie Yeung: An energy boost to brighten my mood   214
"It taught me that hard work and patience pay off and I apply it to all aspects of my life."

50. Sue Cameron: Feeling fabulous helps get us out the door   216
"Being only a novice, I found any sort of training sessions a form of hell and motivating myself to get out the door really tough."

51. Suzie Oswald: I run races with my husband and daughter   217
"More people would run if they took the time to take it easy first."

52. Tara Baumann: Fitness, friendship, enjoyment and challenge   220
"When I run I find myself in a space that I really like to be in."

53. Toni Hackwill: Seeing the social benefits   223
"Running has improved my quality of life. I am happier and I have set goals to train for."

54. Tina Fiegel: An ultra-runner yearns for more   225
"They think I'm doing too much at my age or don't understand that even slow people can do races. But I have running friends."

Acknowledgements

In March 2006 I met Daniel Green, publisher of Australia's Run For Your Life magazine, at an expo held the day before I was set to run the 45-kilometre Six Foot Track trail race in the Blue Mountains in NSW, Australia. Looking to combine my love of running with my professional experience as a journalist and editor, I introduced myself and asked if he was looking for help. He was.

My R4YL briefs were always simple: here's a name and contact details – please write a story. Several of the profiles have turned into cover or feature stories. Each provided me with a little more insight into what it means to be a runner. I thank Daniel for giving me my first opportunity to write about running, which has led to assignments for other endurance sports magazines in Australia and Canada. It also helped inspire the idea for this book.

Running is very personal and unique, yet it's a shared experience too. It's my belief that it is impossible to truly understand what running means to a runner unless you are one. Running allows us to look at ourselves in a different way, to recognise qualities in ourselves that we hadn't before and provide us with the tangible evidence that we possess those qualities.

The majority of women who agreed to answer my questions for this book did not know me and have not met me. We have mostly communicated via email. I was and still am touched by the trust they put in me by sharing some of their deepest thoughts and experiences linked to running.

Running often allows - forces - us to be honest with ourselves and with others. It shows us that we can have our greatest achievements while not looking too pretty in every sense of the word, whether during a tough training session or at a finish line. It is exactly that willingness to put ourselves out there and to bare ourselves that we win our own approval which is sometimes the hardest to gain. We know what it took to get there and we also know where we would have been without having taken the risk.

Running shows us what we are made of, and it proves that we are invariably a lot tougher, more courageous and determined than we give ourselves credit for.

I've worked as a reporter on three different continents since 1996 at the world's top financial newswire, Bloomberg News. I've written thousands of articles and interviewed company CEOs, people managing billions of dollars and central bank officials. My stories have been published in newspapers all over the world. I cherish the experience and opportunities Bloomberg News has given me.

Edward Roussel hired me as an intern reporter for Bloomberg News in Brussels, for which I am grateful. I also thank Martin Cej, then editor for Bloomberg News in Toronto, for recommending my transfer from Belgium to Canada to his boss Kevin Doyle. I don't know what Martin told Kevin but it must have been compelling.

Kevin called me for what I expected to be a gruelling interview about my suitability for the role in Canada. All Kevin asked was, "So you want to move to Canada?" When I confirmed that he said, "Let's make it happen." Kevin, a former Editor of Maclean's magazine, has been one of the most supportive people in my career and I thank him for his belief in me as a journalist and writer. For my subsequent transfer to Australia with Bloomberg News, I thank William Willitts.

Yet for all my experience as a journalist, and later copy-editor at The Australian Financial Review, this is my first book and completing it has been even more challenging that I had imagined. I couldn't help but notice the many similarities between writing a first book and becoming a runner. Many people say they want to take up running but never do. Of those who do try running, many succeed. Many people say they want to write a book but never do. Of those who do start, many succeed. But that didn't make it any easier for me.

The idea of running for an hour can seem like a distant goal when in the beginning every step is tough. The idea of writing a whole book - typically 60,000 words - when you tend to judge every word you write and struggle to find 500 words a day is very daunting too. Articles for Bloomberg News were rarely longer than 800 words while the ones I have written for magazines have not exceeded 3000 words.

You need to find encouragement, inspiration and ask for help. I truly believed that writing a book sharing the knowledge of what running can mean for women's lives would inspire and encourage. But I also had many self-doubts and the ever-looming danger of procrastination.

The first person I asked for help in January 2008 was my running coach Pat Carroll. When I sent him an email explaining my plan and asking if I could interview him and a few of his female clients, I expected he might need a couple of days to consider it. I worried he might question the need for another book on running or my ability to write a book given that it would be my first or that he was already busy enough without being interviewed by a wannabe book author.

I couldn't have been more wrong, and in fact I should have known better. Pat's response reflects his personality as I have come to know him as my coach. He is always positive, especially when I am not, and has a can-do approach without losing sight of reality. He responded to my email immediately, offering all the support I had asked for.

Next I asked several girlfriends who also run if they would be willing to answer questions about their running for this book. Most said yes and did.

The people I had asked for help in any form agreed to do so in the most enthusiastic and positive way. Their responses provided encouragement and inspiration as well as confidence - they believed I could do it for which I am very grateful. I believe it isn't a mere coincidence that runners tend to be very supportive and positive people.

I want to thank all the women who took the time to respond to my questions about their running. You will find all of them in this book and I hope you enjoy reading their stories as much I had writing them. In particular I would like to thank my close friends Fiona Skinner and Gina Unwin for their support and encouragement throughout this process and the many great training sessions we have shared.

Thanks to Elizabeth Bennett, Stacey Harland, Karen Bradley and Karen Scott, none of whom I knew until they responded to my questionnaire for this book. We still have not met, since they live in Australia and I live in Canada, but we are regularly in touch by email and I consider them good friends. Elizabeth has emailed me much-needed encouragement and offered practical advice.

I thank my good friends with whom I have shared many great runs, races and experiences, in particular Stephen Elliott, Anthony Donnelly and Christophe Dumonet.

My friends Charlotte Paul and her husband Kristian Manietta have both encouraged and inspired me in my running. Charlotte was very supportive with this book, at a time when I needed it most.

Pat Carroll has had such a major and positive influence on my running, and therefore my life, since he first began coaching me in June 2005. Since he is based in Brisbane and I lived in Sydney at the time we haven't met that many times. Once he high-fived me as I started the second lap of the Sydney Half Marathon for which he was the MC. He came over to congratulate me after I improved my PB by five minutes in the Canberra marathon. When my partner Tim Moore and I decided to move from Australia, where we had lived for seven years, to Canada I was both excited and sad about that big change. Importantly, I could keep Pat as my running coach and I have. Since arriving in Canada in October 2007 I have set PBs on all the distances I compete in, including improving my 10km time from 41:17 to 39:51. As described above, Pat has been instrumental in this book.

I often think that my grandmother who is now 93 would have made a great distance runner. Her determination is second to none and she is an incredibly strong woman. I am proud to be named after her. She once asked me if I earned money by running. When I told her I have to pay money to race, she said she didn't understand the point of that. Even so, I know she is pleased for me when I do well in a race. My grandmother was especially impressed when I got 35 euros for placing second female in a 10km race in The Netherlands.

My parents Henk and Rezie and my sister Angelique didn't even know about the first running race I did - the 20 kilometres of Brussels in May 1997. I simply hadn't thought of telling them. Most of my races I have done outside of the Netherlands, where I was born, raised and lived until August 1995.

Whenever I race in The Netherlands my parents come to support me, even in pouring rain such as was the case during the first one they watched me do – a 15km road race in 2001. They thought that surely the bad weather meant that I would skip the race. I didn't and their presence spurred me on to finish in a PB (personal best time). The photo my mum took of me shortly after I crossed the finish line then is used as the cover of this book because it captures the happiness of a female distance runner.

My parents and sister even travelled to Frankfurt, Germany, in 2004 to cheer me on for the entire day it takes to race an Ironman triathlon. My sister had in fact come from The Netherlands to Australia to watch me compete in my first Ironman two years earlier. I thank them for supporting me in everything I choose to do.

My biggest supporter is Tim Moore. We have been together for almost nine years. It was our common interest in running and triathlon that had us hang out a lot when we both moved to Sydney, Australia, in 2000. A finisher of nine Ironmans including the Ironman World Championships in Kona, Hawaii, and seven marathons Tim shares my love for endurance sports. It's an important part of our relationship. We also have a career in common. Tim has been a journalist and editor since 1989.

From the moment I first told Tim about my idea for this book until the very end he has been enthusiastic and supportive, even if his encouragement fell on deaf ears at times. I thank him for believing in my ability to complete this book and for sharing my sense of achievement and happiness now that I have done so.

Introduction

Dressed in a cotton T-shirt and a pair of shorts, I put on my shoes – to call them runners would be an exaggeration – and headed out the door. My plan was to run around Centennial Park, a short distance from my house on Eugene Plasky Avenue in Brussels, Belgium. As it turned out, I was a bit optimistic. The five minutes that it took for me to jog the 700 metres to the park was all that my level of fitness could handle. I was OK with that. I couldn't have been any more of a novice. I didn't consider myself a runner, nor did I plan on becoming one. I was motivated to run by two simple objectives – losing weight and improving fitness.

That run was in 1996 when I was 26, and about to complete a post-graduate degree in International and European law before embarking on a new career as a journalist. I also became a runner, although it took me a few years to think of myself that way. Since then both running and writing have shaped my life. Being a runner has taught me many lessons I draw upon as a writer, none more so than that achievements are born in small steps.

Another key lesson is that failure only becomes absolute when we give up. Without true motivation, whatever it may be, we may give in to discomfort or self-doubt before reaching the finish line. But if we can muster self-belief by trusting in our ability, our preparation and our determination, we will achieve what we set out to do.

I may very well have given up on writing this book, my first, if it weren't for my experiences as a runner. Now, living on Canada's west coast, I am training for my 12th marathon which involves covering 42 kilometres and 195 metres. Marathons are completed by simply putting one foot in front of the other, in the same way books are completed word by word; it's about patience and persistence.

While my start as a runner was very basic, I happened upon two crucial points: a strong motivation to run and a willingness to work at it. Over my years of running and in researching this book, I found that many women have a shared experience.

Karen Bradley was 40 when she started running in 2005. Not because she wanted to, but because her best friend and walking partner Stacey did. "I've never been a runner – I didn't like it at all," Karen says. Three years later in 2008, Karen and Stacey finished their first marathon together. And they did their second one in 2009.

In the pages ahead are the stories of how 53 women including Karen and Stacey, ranging in age from 24 to 59, came to be runners and the impact it has had on their lives. Two prominent Australian running coaches - Pat Carroll and Susan Griffith – share some of their expertise about training and motivation.

As with these runners, my reasons for continuing to run are constantly evolving. Fundamentally, I run because it makes me happy. That's why I am a runner – I truly love everything that comes with being one, especially the feelings of independence, self-reliance, freedom, energy, fitness, direction, achievement, self-confidence and self-belief.

Becoming a runner has transformed me mentally, physically and spiritually. Over the years, I have realised running is empowering in the best possible sense of that word. Running has shown me that I can feel confident and in control during tough challenges of my own choosing, such as racing a marathon or writing this book. By being forced to tap into my inner strengths, I have found many that I didn't realise existed. By discovering and honing them through running I have learnt – and am still learning – how to apply them to other aspects of my life.

The fact that you are reading this book means I have fulfilled a goal that I dreamt of for almost two decades. The confidence I found within during my journey as a runner has helped me achieve it. And that is the key inspiration for this book.

Running has changed my life – it is as simple and as profound as that – and I know it has, or can, for many others. I feel strongly about running, and nearly every runner does. So how and what do we feel?

This book focuses on answering that question based on women's experiences because our gender tends to underestimate our ability in sports. While modesty is a beautiful quality, it may also prevent us from recognising our true strengths and accomplishments – and from applying those lessons in other areas of our lives.

Top running coach Susan Griffith often has to remind her runners that the traits they have shown to possess in training can be applied elsewhere. "People tend to box their running. They don't draw the analogies of what they are achieving from their running into the rest of their life until it is brought to their attention. 'You have run a marathon. Why do you think you can't succeed in your job, or have the courage to change jobs?' Think about what you did: the hurdles and strengths you had to pull on in yourself to get to running that marathon. Then draw those strengths into work or your home or whatever."

Family, friends, colleagues and acquaintances alike have often commented on my training discipline yet I rarely do I think about my approach to running along the lines of rules, authority and obedience – those words found in definitions of discipline imply that I have to force myself to run as if I'd rather be doing something else.

The truth is that I always have more and better reasons to go for a run, than not to go. Running makes me feel good in so many ways. It's not hard to make time for the things we enjoy.

That doesn't mean that I am excited about every single run, especially not when it may be cold or raining or I am tired. But I know that I will finish each run feeling better for having done so, for having given my body and mind a chance to relax and having improved my overall sense of wellbeing.

I run because I seek the challenge it provides. Sure, running has become physically easier in some ways the more fit and experienced at it I have become. But there are endless ways to keep testing ourselves from simply making time for it consistently, to running further, faster and on different types of terrain.

Sometimes we need great friends to remind us that we have the strength and ability to accomplish our wildest dreams. Through running I've become one of my own best friends –

instead of being my own worst critic – because it helps me understand that my true potential lies beyond my expectations. I bet my nicest pair of running shoes and most precious finisher's medal that the same goes for you.

Writing this book has challenged my self-belief as few things have. Stringing 90,000 words together in a coherent way has proved more challenging than any of the 11 certified marathons and five Ironman triathlons I've completed. Over the time it took me to complete this project, almost two years, I have run four marathons. In one I set a personal-best time of 3 hours and 7 minutes and in my most recent one I crossed the finish line as the overall female winner.

I relate these two results because they were so far beyond those first few tentative steps in Belgium more than a decade ago. Knowing how far dogged determination can get you is what helped me complete this book.

Running is about testing and challenging our mental and physical boundaries. It takes courage to do so.

CHAPTER 1
That great sense of accomplishment is available to anyone

"It is really important to enjoy the journey rather than feel like it is something you have to do."

Pat Carroll's accomplishments as an elite runner rank him among Australia's top distance runners of all times. Retired from major competition since 2001, Pat has used his love for, and knowledge of, the sport to make the transition to a profession as a running coach. He has been successful from the start and his popularity is growing exponentially every year. Pat has been my coach since June 2005 and I credit him with strengthening my love for running. I like his eternal optimism and encouragement. Pat's guidance has improved my running performance to a level beyond my expectations while keeping injuries at bay.

As a coach, Pat believes in the mental and physical benefits of running available to anyone who is interested. "It gives you a level of fitness that very few other sports can provide. The way you feel about yourself is fantastic. The way you feel in your day-to-day life is great. The fitter you become the more indestructible you feel and that can carry over into your work and your family life. You feel a lot stronger in yourself. Whether you accomplish something in training or whether you accomplish in a race, such as running a 10km, half marathon or a marathon for the first time, it is a sport that is possible for a lot of people and the high that you receive when you have done well is fantastic. I am not saying that that high is any better than for any other sport. The guy who wins a surfing championship or a person who wins the lawn bowls championship or the Australian Open – anything in sport when you win or when you achieve something is just fantastic. But the great thing about running – and I guess triathlon - is that everyone can have their own goals and everyone can walk away feeling incredibly great about themselves because they have just accomplished something, whether it be in training or in competition. It is a natural drug, a natural high."

As a runner, Pat has experienced that sense of achievement many times, especially after finishing his first marathon in 2 hours and 48 minutes. "I crossed the line with tears in my eyes on that day. It was the feeling of achievement; the fact that I'd run 2:48 in my first marathon; that I'd actually finished a marathon; that I'd broken three hours in my first marathon. I went through stages during the race when it was difficult and I managed to overcome that. I guess I was just extremely proud of the fact that I had done it. That first marathon when I crossed the finish line with tears in my eyes is the only time that I've ever been emotional. I've done hundreds of races and I've won hundreds of races but that first marathon was the only time I was emotional when I crossed the line. I ended up running my fastest marathon later in 2:09 and I didn't have tears in my eyes that day, though I still felt bloody fantastic about what I'd just done. What I am saying is that the natural high doesn't discriminate - regardless of the pace it carries over throughout everyone in the whole event."

Running goals don't need to involve races. "If people don't want to be involved in competition then they can get themselves a goal in training. Maybe they are going further in their own training run than they have ever done before. When they get home and they say to their husband or their wife that they just ran to so-and-so and back, they feel really good about themselves because they have accomplished something they had never done before. One of the main benefits is that incredible sense of achievement that is available to everyone. That's a great positive with running: feeling good about yourself because you can achieve a goal. It is really important in life that you feel good about yourself and running can certainly provide that."

Pat provides guidance by writing training programs he develops for each runner individually, based on their fitness level and goals. He coaches runners who live close enough to attend Pat Carroll Running Group (PCRG) training sessions as well as people like me who live elsewhere and do his training sessions alone.

PCRG is popular and increasingly so. A recent Tuesday session drew 153 runners – about a year ago that was the average amount of people who would show up for an entire week's three sessions. PCRG meets on Tuesday, Thursdays and Fridays. While the rising attendance at PCRG has a lot to do with Pat's skills as a coach, it is also indicative of a growing interest in the sport. "I have noticed the increase in popularity of running in general."

About 60 percent of the runners in his group are female. His group has grown mainly through word of mouth. "The best form of marketing, I have found, is if you provide a good service and people talk to other people. It just flows from there."

Pat guides runners who vary in age and ability – but they all share the desire to focus on a goal. About 80 per cent of the people who attend his group are aged 30 or older. "I deal with every-day people who wish to accomplish something."

That goal may be to run their first marathon or it may be to better a previous marathon time. "Probably 90 percent of the people I deal with are goal driven. The main reason they come to someone like me is because they want direction so that they can improve. They all have a similar personality I guess. I get more of a feel for their personality in my group than for my online clients. The people in my group are successful in their work and running provides a huge balance in their lives. They're positive, friendly and social people. There are very few introverts in my running group. Very seldom will I get quiet achievers coming along who just do their own thing and go home. Everyone gets involved in the whole group thing."

Pat highly recommends any runner to train with a group, regardless of whether it is led by a coach. People may be encouraged by getting involved with other runners who are at a similar level of fitness and speed. "The group environment is a fantastic way to get involved in running. It's like riding a bike or riding a horse - once you have done it you will realise you can do it. When people who have never run in a running group before come along to PCRG they are 100 percent impressed. They always come back. They think, 'Man this is unbelievable: all these people, all goal-driven and all running hard in a session. Everyone is positive and supportive'. So people think this is fantastic and they do come back."

The social aspect is important to the people who train with Pat's group. "Whether all running groups are the same I don't know, but with my running group it's very social. Afterwards, everyone is standing around for a good 15 minutes having a chat. It's outdoors, it's social and it offers a lot more than what the gym does which would be a main competitor to a running group."

PCRG runners are judged by the effort they put into their runs, rather than by their absolute speed. "I do have people in my group who take 16 minutes to run 3 km flat to the boards. So these people take 5 ½ minutes to run 1km. That's not out of reach for most people once they get involved in running. If you can bowl along at 5:30/km pace reasonably comfortably, you'll fit in OK."

Many people who ask Pat for guidance in their running have done run training before, though not necessarily with a coach. When people are just starting out with running, Pat advises them to follow a very basic walking/running program. "Run for 2 minutes and walk for 2 minutes, or something like that. It depends what level of fitness they are at but they should walk and run. They can gradually increase the time they run and reduce the time they walk."

While Pat will encourage anyone who is interested in running, he believes the sport is not for everyone - and that's OK. "You're either a runner or you are not. It's not something you can make yourself be. If you are a runner, then you are going to be running pretty much most of your life. You might run once every couple of weeks or you might run once a week or something, and then you might eventually get more into it. They are the people that I deal with. People who have always dabbled in it here and there but eventually finally want to give it a go, or finally want to run a marathon. If people come to me and say, 'I've never run a step in my life', then I know when I send them some sort of training over the internet that they are probably not going to carry on with it. They haven't become a runner by themselves. Running has really got to be part of you. It has to be part of your character or something that you enjoy, rather than, 'I want to do a marathon or a half marathon so I'd better start running'," says Pat.

People who have little experience with running often haven't thought about how they are going make time to do their training and the commitment that it requires. Pat says it is crucial to do so. "If you are going to set yourself a challenge in running, then obviously you are going to step up your preparation and do more than what you have done previously. Before you do, it's very important to step back and ask yourself whether you are actually going to commit to this. It's a matter of structuring your training times around other things that are happening in your life.

"You have to work out the times of the week, and the times of the day that will ensure you are going to get out the door and that nothing is going to stand in your way. One female online client in Townsville wanted to train for the Gold Coast marathon and we decided her long run would be on Saturday morning. Then she emailed me saying she had found a running buddy and they were going to do their long run on a Thursday evening. I told her that it wasn't going to work. No one in this world is going to head out the door at 5pm for a three-hour training run in 35-degree [Celsius or 95-degree Fahrenheit] heat after you've been working during the day. If you structure your training like that, then it is not going to happen. You're going to have holes all over the joint with regards to training that you have missed because it was too hot or you were too tired after a day's work."

Pat strongly advised her to do her long runs early. "An hour and a half in the evening is not out of the question after you have been working during the day. But imagine being at work and thinking that after work you have got a three-hour training run. You'd feel like you are carrying bricks all day. You just can't beat the freshness of the morning for running. Only a small percentage of people do prefer the evening but the vast majority would be morning runners. It's fresh, you feel alive, you've got lots of energy, you know that it's your opportunity to get out the door and get it done. If you leave it for the evening you go through the day feeling burdened because you haven't done it and it is waiting for you at the end of the day, rather than feeling energised because you worked out in the morning."

People who are more experienced runners have often already learnt how to make a commitment to their training. Pat estimates that about 90 percent of the more seasoned runners who ask him for a training program will stick to it. "I'd get 10 percent of people who are already runners and wishing to improve that I won't hear from again. A strong percentage of people do carry through with the training I set and correspond with me throughout. Obviously I get the odd ones who fall by the wayside through injury or illness."

Pat often has to tell his runners to do less training and to run less often. This is especially the case for female clients, he has found. "Possibly women are more inclined to do more than what they should. Women are more inclined to get carried away with their enthusiasm which is normally their undoing. They possibly tend to be more on the compulsive side. I have seen a great deal more women fall by the wayside through running because they just train hard too many days in a row. They go for training runs with groups on the weekend that are too quick for them, so they are running pretty much close to their half-marathon best pace to keep up with the group. If you do that week in week out, you come undone. They think, 'If I do more I am going to feel better' or 'If I do more then I am going to improve more'. You really can't go past the fact that you can only take on what your body can physically handle. There's only a certain workload that people can take on depending on how many years they have been involved. If you do too much, then you are going to fall apart with injuries like stress fractures and so on."

Pat says his online clients usually seek his guidance for three key reasons. "One, to get direction because they have absolutely no idea what to do; two, you get people who want just to be answerable to me to help with their motivation - another reason not to sleep in; and then you have got people who have no problems with motivation but who are goal-driven and want to improve."

While Pat will devise the best training program for each runner based on their experience and goals, he makes no promises when it comes to results. He also warns against coaches who do offer guarantees on finishing times or running a marathon in three months. "I never give a guarantee. I will send a training program which I am confident would be a sensible path to follow, but I won't guarantee. People have to realise that some people improve faster than others. Injury is always there. You can't deny that and there is no guarantee that you are going to improve. I look at it as more of a journey. If you want to have someone to correspond with and offer you a sensible path, then I can offer that."

He recommends anyone seeking out a coach to make sure that this person has experience in running themselves, though not necessarily as an elite athlete. "It's important that it is someone who has been involved in running, maybe not at the top end but definitely a runner. If you have never run a day in your life and you have no experience in running, then how do you know what a 21km effort feels like? I have seen coaches who have never run and have absolutely totally smashed runners as a result of that because they don't know what the human body can actually handle. That's a very important part of coaching in running. Because running is such a stressful action to put your body under, you really have to understand and get a feel for where the person is at, their level of development and what they are going to be able to handle without falling apart. So you are after a sensible coach who has been a runner or is a runner."

Pat always stresses the importance of recovery in training, something that often surprises his clients at first, especially if they do or have done triathlons which consist of swimming, cycling and running. "When they deal with me, people become more aware of the importance of recovery. You get a lot of people these days who are involved in triathlon and I think that killed the importance of recovery. They do so many things with the bike and the swims: it's possible to involve multiple consecutive hard days in the pool and on the bike - however you can't do the same with running. Running is different. One of the main advantages of dealing with me, and I instil this in people all the time, is that I tell them to back off a little bit. OK you have got to train hard but look at what you're doing when you are training hard. You are breaking your body down and your body needs to rebuild. And if you smash yourself again too soon, you are going to enter your next run feeling tired or sore because you haven't given yourself enough time to recover. That's one thing with running that is totally different with cycling – you just need to respect your body's necessity to repair and rebuild before you move on."

Budding marathoners often think that they need to cover the 42.915-kilometre race distance in training first. Pat tells them no, time and again. "They don't have to run incredibly long in training, just because they have never run a marathon before or because their marathon is going to take them 4 hours or 5 hours. I'm often like a stuck record but I tell these people to just keep churning through 3-hour training runs. OK, it's going to take you 4 or 5 hours on the day. If a climber's mission is to climb Mt Everest, they don't go and climb Everest to prepare. They may climb a mountain that is maybe three-quarters the height a few times but Everest is the thing they finally are going to conquer. There is no difference with regards to the marathon: you don't run 42km in training to prepare yourself for the 42km. You involve multiple 30km runs on a weekly basis. You do that a number of times just like the guy who climbs the mountain three-quarter the height of Everest a number of times to prepare for his summit."

Pat says the same principle applies for the half marathon if you have never raced this distance before. "It is more like looking at it from a realistic point of view. It's often very easy to be on the outside looking in as a coach. Sometimes runners feel that they have to prove to themselves in training that they can do it - rather than having faith in a long and healthy campaign."

Pat says it is very important to prepare properly by increasing race distances gradually to allow the body to adapt to the stresses of running farther distances. "I don't hold back if someone approaches me and says, 'I've run a couple of 10km races. The most I've run is an hour. I want to run a marathon in 12 weeks from now. Can you help me?' And I'll say, 'No, go for the half marathon'."

Pat adds that his partner Susan doesn't follow his guidance and proves to be the exception to his rules. "Susan runs the Gold Coast marathon every year. And she's a mess when she finishes it. She often has a limited campaign, however she regularly takes part in aerobics and she also cycles. Sue is a bit of an enigma because her theory is: A marathon is easy if you train for it. It's a real challenge if you don't."

CHAPTER 2
Exercise is one of the critical elements to a person's wellbeing

"People who take running up later in life find that it gives them a level of confidence they didn't know existed."

Susan Griffith began running at an early age, initially as a way to improve her fitness for other sports she played competitively - hockey and squash. Then she focused on running as a sport, before making it her profession as a coach. Now 47, she guides both individuals and groups, and often leads workshops on running. "Running has been a huge part of my life over the last 23 years. It provides me with a skill and talent now as a coach where I can impart my knowledge on to others to help them achieve their goals. I really enjoy that. Running has always been a part of my life and I am consistently blown away by the fact that people who take it up later in life find that it gives them a level of confidence they didn't know existed. I feel privileged to have had those benefits all my life," she says.

Don't tell Susan that you cannot run because she will likely disagree with you. "Unless you have a physical disability that is going to stop you running you can run. The question is: do you want to run? There are a few people that for whatever reason can't run. They may have some joint problems. My husband, for example, had a knee reconstruction done poorly after a rugby incident when he was in high school. But most people can run if they want to."

And that's the key: finding reasons and ways to enjoy your running so that you wish to make it a part of your life. Being a runner is a lifestyle for Susan, something she chooses to do because she likes it. "It's hard for those people who start running because they know they have to get fit or lose weight but they don't really enjoy it. They should find something they do enjoy - otherwise it's a chore and not a lifestyle," Susan says.

As a coach, she often recommends others to take up running. She teaches a six-week Learn to Run course and has done so for more than 15 years. This clinic is especially popular with women. While she has coached plenty of male runners, about 80 percent in her beginners' courses are female. Creating a safe, comfortable and encouraging learning environment is very important. "This course is to help women who want to give running a go but who are afraid of all the things that go along with it. They may be afraid of going outside and being exposed, to be looked at by men in particular and having sexist comments made to them. Afraid of the gear they may have to wear, like small shorts or whatever. Afraid that they are going to be laughed at, that they can't keep up or can't do it and that they'll fail. They find the whole thing intimidating but somewhere along the line someone has encouraged them or suggested they come to a beginners' course. I try to make them feel safe, explain that becoming a runner is a journey and that we will take it in small sections. I tell them that it is OK to walk and jog to start with - that is normal for most people."

Susan has seen big transformations take place in this clinic. Many beginners can't run 100 metres when they start the course and are amazed at their improvement in less than two months. "I see them often shocked that they are able to run 3km or 4km without stopping by the end of week six. At the start of the clinic they never believed they could do it. That's the most powerful thing that happens."

Susan often discusses motivation, especially when beginners express doubts about their ability to do the training. "When people start and say, 'This is hard. I don't know if I can do this,' I try to find out what their motivation is to start running. You will get various answers obviously. Some people say, 'I used to run when I was at school and I really enjoyed it'. Some will say, 'My husband wants me to run because he runs'. Most people say, 'Because I want to lose weight'."

Once Susan understands their primary reason to run, she helps them to set their goals accordingly. For example if the goal is to lose a certain amount of weight, she discusses how running fits into that picture as well as other things the runner can do to achieve the goal weight and maintain it. "I also encourage them to talk to other runners. That's why I think the groups are really good. They can come and share experiences and find out that they are not Robin Crusoe. Most people find it difficult to get their gear on and get out on their own or that it hurts a bit," she says.

Susan says she always encourages her beginning runners to focus on what goes well in each training session. "Try to find out what was good about your run. Was there any stage where you felt good, and try to focus on the positive elements about it. And they might say, 'Yes when I finished I felt good'."

Susan also discusses running equipment such as shoes, bras, socks and other clothing. She points out potential hazards like blisters and chafing. "You can read about these sorts of things but having a chat woman on woman seems more comforting. By the end of week six they have usually bought a new bra top or gear that might be a little bit more risqué than the long pants that they wore initially. They may have ventured into wearing some board shorts-type things or into trying out new materials like Coolmax, instead of wearing a cotton T-shirt. So they start to have some tools that allow them to explore. It feels better to run in a proper top or to have proper running shoes as opposed to the old cross-trainers that have been batting about the house for a couple of years. You see them more confident about themselves and their interaction to others."

Susan says her role as a coach extends beyond running. She is often asked for advice on nutrition and often discusses topics that have nothing to do with exercise. "You don't just talk about running when you go out for an hour with people. You end up talking about your whole life."

Running can change lives in many ways, Susan says. Sometimes it forces novice runners to alter their social life, especially for women in their 20s. "They tell me, 'It's really hard because my friends want me to go out drinking with them on Friday night and I don't want to go because I want to get up and run with the running club at 7:30am on Saturday morning. I can't do both'," she says.

Susan tells them to change friends, often to her clients' surprise. She is not kidding. "I say, 'You want to do this, they want to do that. How much do you want to run in the morning? Really you want to run. You best come to an agreement with them about your life now or try to persuade them to come along. But if this is the way you want to go, you have to do something about your relationship with these people for you to achieve what you want to do'."

Becoming a runner will often lead to a transformation in self-image, especially if a person begins with the goal to lose excess kilograms. "From a health perspective, obviously the people who are overweight when they start running can recreate their body shape and that can be life-changing. And a lot of women wouldn't know that they could run, so that can be life-changing," Susan says.

Novice runners who go on to reach goals such as finishing a half marathon or a marathon start applying the lessons from their accomplishments to the rest of their life, their career and their family. The resulting increase in self-confidence is usually a positive though it may also cause dramatic changes. "In the main I think the pluses definitely outweigh the minuses. But I have also seen marriages break down because of it. Now whether those marriages were good or healthy relationships in the first place I don't know. People might say, 'Yes it was the best thing I did - my husband left because I'd become this boring runner'. Or, 'My wife left me because I decided I want to run a marathon twice a year'. Changes can be in all shapes and sizes. Over years of running and coaching you see a lot and a lot of changes that do occur in people through running."

Susan often finds herself reminding runners of the strength they have shown through their training and racing, and their opportunity and ability to apply that in other areas. "People tend to box their running. They don't draw the analogies of what they are achieving from their running into the rest of their life until it is brought to their attention. You have run a marathon. Why do you think you can't succeed in your job or have the courage to change jobs? Think about the strengths you had to pull on in yourself to get to running that marathon and draw those strengths into work, your home or whatever."

Susan says runners usually come to her through word of mouth. She says she finds runners reluctant to pay for a training program. "They will go to a personal trainer and they will spend hundreds of dollars on physiotherapy, garments and heart rate monitors. There is a tradition in athletics that things are for free. I think the industry itself, a lot of people, put a lot into running and will do it for free because they love it. And that's fine but when you are a coach you have to pay to get trained, you have to pay for your insurance every year, every three years you have to renew your credentials and you have to go on training courses on various things to get your points up to keep accredited. So a coach will incur a lot of direct and indirect expenses. If someone wants a program then you've have got to spend the time talking to them, assessing their needs, writing the program, and explaining the program and supporting them through it. So there is a costing."

Having a coach design a training program for an athlete specifically will optimise their performance, she says. "I design a program to meet their needs and requirements. I design around when they can train to fit it in with their lives. It makes them accountable. It helps them to take realistic steps towards their goal. It is a safer way to train. It is also education because they learn about periodisation: why we have weeks with a heavier training load and those with lower ones, why you need recovery runs and why you don't play catch-up if you've been sick or injured. It is a learning process for them. When I coach somebody I'd like to think that they come out better informed at the end of the program so they can be self-sufficient."

Susan warns runners against following a training program created for someone else to save the expense of getting a personalised one. "If I am writing a program for John and his mate Neil says he'll just do what John does, then that could be a big problem. It is unlikely that their running history, training tolerances, time availability and ability are the same. So why do they think their training programs should be the same? I think a lot of people spend a lot of time running on either somebody else's program or a generic program from a magazine. Three years down the track they come and say, 'You know I just don't seem to be getting any better'. When you have got a coach there to support you, it helps to keep you focused and reminds you that you shouldn't whack that extra 20km in the next week or that you won't be good to run with an injury or a virus."

Susan especially cautions beginning runners against the temptation to log too many miles in training or racing. She recommends novice runners limit themselves to a 10km race, definitely in the first six months of their training. "Personally I wouldn't promote that new runners try to do long distances in their first 12 months of running. Lots of people say, 'It is fantastic - I did a half marathon'. But what you don't hear about is, 'I haven't been able to run for three months as I have been injured because of it'. Stress fractures and strains are risks for runners who increase their volume of running too much too soon."

Susan says that the jump from training for and racing a 10km to a half marathon is big. Unfortunately few races offer an option in between these two. "Running races could do with a midway standard distance between the 10km and 21km – say 16km. This would help people to gain relevant experience and to get strong before they start to load on the kilometres towards a half marathon."

In training Susan has her runners aiming to run for a certain time, say one hour, rather than a certain distance, say 12km. Still people in her running groups always want to know how far they ran in their sessions. "I tell them not to worry so much about the distance - it's the time that matters. Even now with the group I take on Tuesday nights - they have been running for a year - all of them want to know how far they ran in a session. One of the guys in the group has a Garmin and he always has got the distance. He runs a bit further because he's faster so I send him off on loops. He'll say, 'I did 8.5km' and so I'll say, 'We probably have done 7.5km so put it in your log then."

She highly recommends every runner looks after their body with regular stretching and massages, something she has learned the hard way. When she took up running more than two decades ago, stretching wasn't part of training programs. "I had injury problems through running for too many years without stretching. I strongly recommend people stretch and go to yoga if they can because that gives you a core strength and stability.

Certain types of yoga definitely do. I have been an advocate now of Power Yoga which is very strong flowing yoga. It's the first time I have found a yoga that I can do because it moves. Being a runner I found previously that yoga was too static and hummy."

Susan recommends runners get a massage once a month if it fits in their budget. "It should be a total body massage because with a lot of running-related injuries you think it is your hamstrings but the reality is that it might be your lower back. So if you just have a massage on your legs, it might be missing the critical point that will release."

For Susan, running had long been a way to take care of her fitness for other sports. In 1986 she changed her focus. "I started fun-running as I wanted to do something challenging that I wasn't very good at. I had played State I grade squash for a number of years and that was highly competitive. A sport where I wasn't expected to win was more relaxing."

These days Susan alternates running, cycling and yoga. She believes it is very important to keep her body in balance to prevent injuries. She consistently runs three times a week. While she doesn't get hung up about going for a run, she also doesn't like foregoing her sports especially not for a few days in a row. "If I don't run or exercise I feel less energised, both mentally and physically. I long to get back into it and I feel unhappy about having to miss my exercise."

A run always lifts Susan's spirits. While she believes in great runs, of which she has had many, she doesn't in bad ones. "When I've had a great run I feel very energised, satisfied and ready to tackle whatever is thrown at me. There is rarely a bad run. Every run serves its purpose – you run, you learn, you move on. I rarely feel unhappy about my run. It is what it is, I don't analyse it too much. There are days when I run and it just feels easy, and there are other days when there are a few aches and pains. So a good run is determined by doing the whole distance, whatever that is, and not feeling any physical pain at the end."

She'll run regardless of her mood. "Mood doesn't make a difference. I run when it fits in with the rest of my schedule. When I am in a training program, or even when I am not, I sometimes skip sessions. Work, weather and family are the main reasons. If the reason is out of my control then I don't feel guilty. If I am following a training program and am just being lazy then I'd feel guilty for a while but it's my decision, no one else's, so I have to justify it to myself and live with it."

Susan says she doesn't reward herself for consistent training or reaching certain goals. "I guess I don't worry so much about what I eat when I am consistently training; I have to reduce what I eat if I don't exercise."

The people close to Susan are supportive of her passion and she believes they also understand what running means to her. "They understand it's just a part of who I am. Because I have always participated in sport my family, friends and husband don't give it a second thought – it's just what I do."

Susan no longer feels competitive. "In my early running days I always tried to do the best I could, although I was never going to be a champion. Nowadays I run for fun and the health benefits and am not competitive. I am very focused in other areas of my life and like to do the best I can. With running I feel been-there-done-that – there's no need to keep trying to prove myself. I would rather help others achieve their goals."

She appreciates the health benefits of running. "Running is important to my health but not the be all and end all. I understand that I have been running for a long time and I know that as I get older it is more difficult to put in the kilometres I used to. I do not have the slight figure of a runner and so there has been a heavy load through my body over the years. Yes there are lots of health benefits but I believe running for most adults should be done in conjunction with other exercise, for example cycling, swimming, yoga or hiking. I am healthy because I exercise - running is just one form of exercise I do. I have had periods of not running due to injury during which I cycled and was still healthy then."

By the same token, her self-esteem and self-image have been affected by exercise in general. "Running in itself isn't that important to my self-esteem and self-image but exercise is. My profession is in health and wellness and I believe that exercise is one of the critical elements to a person's wellbeing."

CHAPTER 3
Running makes me happy
"I have three small children, work four days a week, and can honestly say running is my release."

In January 2007 Angela Adamson decided it was time to get off the treadmill and start running outside. The mother of three joined the Pat Carroll Running Group. "I knew that I could run. I had done treadmill work at the local gym on and off for around four years. I am a very determined and highly motivated person who seems to push herself in everything that she does. I just wanted to make that next step and get on the road," Angela says.

Angela took that step and then some - a year later the 33-year-old started training for the Gold Coast marathon. "Running has become rather addictive. My goals are constantly changing from running 10km, to running a half marathon and now a marathon. What's next?"

Like many running mothers, Angela enjoys the time she spends training because it recharges her batteries. Occasionally she wonders if it is a selfish pursuit but she knows her family benefits too. "Running is a major part of my life. It helps me keep fit and healthy. It is me-time. I am away from all those stresses in life. I don't have to think about work, family, home - I just focus on me. Sometimes I think it is a bit selfish but then I realise that as long as the balance is right I am happy - which in turn makes for happy children and happy hubby. I think I am a lot calmer, more patient and less resentful when dealing with the children. I really enjoy the time with them - I feel I can give them 100 percent of me. Running gives me energy to chase my little ones. It helps me mentally to stay focused and enjoy life."

Angela's husband Doug trains with the same running group as she does, so they alternate their days of training. With Angela and Doug both committed to their running lifestyles, they make time in their busy schedules by getting up early as it takes them 45 minutes to get to the group's meeting point. "I work four full days a week and have three children under the age of six. My husband is totally supportive as he understands being a runner himself. The children just think it is a normal part of our lives. Certain family and friends think we are mad and give that crazy look when we have to leave a BBQ early because we are up early for a long run. My husband's parents - although they live a few hours away - help out whenever they can so that we can get a long run in together or participate in a major event."

Doug's own passion for running means that he understands hers, particularly when an injury sidelined Angela. "I injured my groin and couldn't run for a few months. I was devastated. My husband felt so guilty for doing his runs and would often just not talk to me about the run because he knew how bad I was feeling. We sometimes take it all for granted. It takes an injury to realise that. It made me more motivated to stay fit. My main concern was losing my overall fitness, so I pursued other areas such as pool running," Angela says.

But when they are both running well and racing, they are competitors first and foremost. "Hell yes. Ask my husband - we are competitive all the time. We both did the Noosa half marathon and [our coach] Pat [Carroll] was on the loud speaker commentating. I finished about a minute before my husband. Pat told the crowd on loud speaker, 'This is Doug everyone - his wife has just beaten him. How does it feel Doug?' A proud moment in my running career, probably one Doug would like to forget. I am sure he will get his own back."

Angela runs four times a week. She's on a training program with Pat for the Gold Coast marathon. She keeps track of all the sessions she does. While some people enjoy a training program because it keeps them motivated to do their runs, Angela has one to avoid doing too much. "Because I consider myself as highly motivated - probably too motivated - I wanted a sensible program that will hopefully prevent me from overdoing things and getting injured."

She enjoys training with PCRG because it is a great way to socialise and be inspired by other runners. "I enjoy running in a group because this is where I have met some of the most inspirational people. In a group it seems to be more motivating and I can guarantee that if I had done a similar run on my own I may have given up a lot earlier. I like getting to know more about fellow runners. You learn so much from them and their experiences."

The social aspect of group running is important but not essential, Angela says, adding that the main purpose remains doing her training. She does other sports but only to advance her running. "I am a runner and only a runner. I have to pursue other areas such as Pilates and swimming - I am hoping it will improve my posture and strength to become a better runner."

On a great run Angela feels empowered and confident. "If I have a great run, it can boost my mood for that day. It puts a spring in my step and I have a sense of achievement. I feel that it is more mental than physical. Once you put your mind to it you can do anything. I run no matter what mood I am in. It is a way of life."

Running has changed her life in the sense that it has made her more disciplined, determined and energetic, Angela says. "I also have a greater appreciation for life - running along the Brisbane River, taking in the sights, breathing in the fresh air and feeling the sun. I have met some great people. It has given me a greater awareness of my body mentally and physically. Overall, it has made me a better person – a good mum and a good wife … when we are not competing."

Angela enjoys the health benefits that come with being fit, though says that running alone is not a guarantee for physical wellness. "When pushing your body to its limit and seeing the improvements from week to week it must be important to your health. I think that you can be fit but not necessarily healthy if you have an unbalanced lifestyle such as eating wrong foods."

She has recommended running to friends and colleagues, saying that all it takes to convince them are her experiences. "They just hear my running stories and think if a mum of three can do it – anyone can."

Angela says running has given her more confidence, therefore greater self-esteem. Her main motivation to run is because she enjoys it. "Running makes me happy."

CHAPTER 4
Taking care of yourself is not selfish
"Cool wind in my hair on a hot afternoon, boosts of unexpected energy, and positive, unsolicited comments from people I least expect"

Anne-Maree Jaggs, 46, began running in November 2007 because she wanted to get fit. Restraints on her time and budget made running the best option. And, besides, she was inspired by her partner Judy. "Judy has been running for about 10 years but the last three seriously - for herself. She only entered her first fun runs in 2007. She runs on her own and designs her own training programs. I want to feel and look as good as she does. And have her stamina," Anne-Maree says.

She says Judy has been very supportive of her running ambitions. As a new runner, Anne-Maree's 2007 Christmas presents included a running log book and a voucher to sign up for a one-month online training program with Pat Carroll. Anne-Maree says knowing that she has to report back to her running coach at the end of the week as to whether she did her training sessions inspires her to complete them. "I am the kind of person who needs to report to another," she says. She also enjoys filling out her log book as she finds that keeping track of the kilometres she has covered on foot is an excellent motivational tool.

Anne-Maree's desire to improve her health was and still is her main motivation for her new running lifestyle. "I think about the health benefits all the time. At my age and carrying too much weight, it was the right decision to make. I am aware that I need to take better care of my eating habits, but that running is one of the best aerobic activities for me."

Like many people, Anne-Maree had difficulty finding time for her new activity with a full-time job and two small children. But she decided that making running a priority would provide benefits for herself – and her family – that far outweighed the challenges of fitting it into her already busy life.

And naturally Judy is a very supportive partner because of her own running passion. "She is very proud of me," Anne-Maree says.

Now Anne-Maree runs four days a week while Judy trains four to five days a week. "We agreed early on that she'd do a morning run and I'd run early evening," says Anne-Maree, who varies the days but not the amount of sessions over the week. Judy isn't the only one encouraging Anne-Maree's newfound love of running. "Family and friends are very, very happy and supportive. So are neighbours and people on my bus who see me. Our kids accept that we need to go out for a run."

She has also discovered the encouraging nature of other pedestrians, both runners and walkers alike. "I am a solo runner but I run around the local streets and get a buzz seeing other runners and walkers, and smiling in support for each other."

When Anne-Maree found an activity she liked, she made a commitment to spend the time and effort needed, enlisted a professional coach and followed his advice. And six months after she took up running, Anne-Maree finished her first fun run, which was a 4½-kilometre female-only race, with great success. "I hurt, I mainly ran, and managed to do the 4.5km run in 20-odd minutes. What a buzz. One of the best parts was towards the end of the run. We were running past the massive pink tide of walkers just starting out on their walk and I was thinking, `Hell, I'm actually running - how cool is that.' I used to be just a walker and didn't think I could ever change. It was fun and really motivating, with lots of women laughing and enjoying themselves and feeling pretty proud of their achievements."

Her commitment to running has brought about a big mental shift. "There are two ways that running has been a turning point in my life. One is that I've always done things for other people - putting others first in the hope they'd like me. I seem to have that sort of personality. If it means not doing what makes me happy or is best for my health, I can be easily swayed, plus I'd rather not argue. The second is the fat-word. I've yo-yoed with my weight all my life, and am quite frankly nervous about looking great. Stupid as that sounds, people treat jolly fat people differently to skinny people. Slim is power? Hell, what could happen? Running is the first thing I have been able to tell myself that I need and must do, and can enjoy. It has flexibility in terms of when and where I run, and if I choose to run with others. I'm chuffed with myself for making this healthy activity part of my life. I intend to run and jog for as many years as I can."

Anne-Maree has learnt that each run is different. Sometimes she feels great, sometimes she doesn't. "On a great run, I feel a bit euphoric and my body is buzzy."

She has also found that the feeling of whether she had a great run or a not-so-great run often depends on her frame of mind. On days when her training feels tough, Anne-Maree says she accepts it and tells herself that at least she's out there walking and running. "It reminds me to stay with it as I am a learner, and that there will always be good and bad days for everything. The discipline keeps me going. I don't get upset, as I'm not competing."

Anne-Maree has also accepted that patience is a virtue when it comes to improving fitness. "I am a competitive person by nature, and tend to overdo exercise when I get going. I am learning to hold back, not push for speed but run for longer."

The single-most important thing about running for Anne-Maree is that she is doing something for herself that benefits her family as well. "It's for me and no one else. It's the only selfish thing I do. But is it selfish to take care of yourself? I think women do put their families first, to the detriment of their own health. I now know why my partner comes back from a run smiling - I used to think she looked a bit mad."

CHAPTER 5
Running my first marathon was incredible
"You end up with some hyperventilating guy slapping around behind you and you slow down so you don't have to call an ambulance."

This 31-year-old, who wants to remain anonymous, began running at the age of 26. She gradually built up her stamina by alternating walking and running until she was able to do a half-hour jog. Initially her primary motivation was to maintain her fitness after moving to Australia from abroad. "My first real run was a 10km in March 2003 as part of a work triathlon team. I had previously done a lot of outdoors activities like mountain biking and bush walking. Then I moved to Australia where I was too scared of snakes and all the other wildlife to venture into the bush on my own and didn't have anyone to do this with. In an attempt to keep fit enough to enjoy those activities when I caught up with friends and family, I decided to try running along local suburban streets, something I felt happy enough to do on my own."

Now she still runs to keep up her level of fitness but also for the sheer enjoyment she experiences. She loves challenging herself to run further or faster and prepares for specific running events. Running means many things to her. "A sense of freedom and enjoying the outdoors. Escape from the pressures of life. Exhilaration from feeling your lungs stretched to their limits. A feeling of satisfaction when you run to exhaustion. Time to think and space to breathe."

While she loves running, she says it isn't her favourite sport. "It's hard to say. To me, running is a solitary sport: I started doing it by myself and my friends still don't include any keen runners. I enjoy running for the solitude I can achieve but I enjoy other activities for the companionship I have with them. It's nice to have a balance. Physically, I find running more enjoyable than road cycling or mountain biking and it is more efficient as it takes less time to feel like you've had a decent effort. But then again I started running in Brisbane where we are spoiled with fantastic weather so while riding or mountain biking or hiking in terrible weather never bothered me, I can't bring myself to run in it."

She enjoys the flexibility of running. "I go through periods where I do a lot of travel for work so running is much easier to take with you than for example cycling. It's a good way to explore the local streets and parks before work and helps you to wake up and feel refreshed for what is usually a long day ahead."

She runs four times a week on average. "This is reasonably consistent but has dropped to once per week when I am training for something else, like a major cycling event, or when I am on a multi-day hike. It increases to five days per week if I am preparing for a running event like a marathon."

She has been keeping a training diary for the past four years listing all the types of exercise she does. "I started only to remember what I had done and to make sure that I wasn't overdoing anything and was eating enough to balance activity levels. I have just begun a specific running log this year in an attempt to put more effort into running so we will see how that goes."

She is a morning runner because of the climate, though not by nature which proves challenging at times. "I live in Brisbane where it's generally too hot to run in the middle of the day so you have to get up quite early to run or else wait until the evening when it is dark. Unfortunately I am not a morning person so I do struggle sometimes with fitting running into my life. The snooze button on my alarm is a bad thing."

She initially found little support or interest for her running. "Nobody really paid any attention to my morning jogs until I started entering fun runs and doing reasonably well for a recreational runner. Then they showed supportive interest. But when I said I was going to try to run a marathon, again there was a feeling of not being taken too seriously."

Her performance in the marathon surprised many as she finished in a very swift 3 hours and 4 minutes. "I pick up distance much more easily than speed so my marathon time was just over half-marathon pace. People were shocked I think because it was so close to the elusive three hours that many go on about. Also, colleagues of my family who are very serious about training for Ironman events and the like said that they couldn't run that distance in that time. Most of these are quite fit guys who've been running for a lot longer than me.

"That and the fact that my helpful brother started rumours that a marathon is supposed to be the physical limit of what people can do - this scared me as he is an extreme climber and certainly knows about limits so I nearly pulled out. Then I read an article that said that 250,000 Americans run a marathon every year so I thought that if that many people can run a marathon then I should be able to. My brother's rumours had got a few people worried so I had a lot of anxious phone calls after the first marathon with people expecting me to be on my death bed."

Her impressive marathon performance boosted the support by friends and family for her running. While that was welcome it has unfortunately also brought an unwelcome side effect. "Now there is a very keen interest by friends and family as to how my running is going and when am I doing another race. It actually reached the stage of too much pressure last year when work and travel commitments meant I couldn't do as much running as I would have liked. I think the few races I did enter disappointed a few people."

She says that family and friends probably do not understand what running means to her. "A few friends are a bit resentful when I don't go riding with them because I want to get a run in. I think a few people are shocked to hear what time I manage to get out of bed some mornings."

That first marathon is still her most cherished experience involving running. "I had trained well and was happy to be there and see if I could do it. Everything went perfectly – fantastic scenery, beautiful day and a fantastic group of onlookers. I enjoyed the entire run and did better than I had hoped."

During and after a great run she feels exhilarated. "Awake and full of positive energy to start the day. Physically exhausted and mentally invigorated. Grinning on the inside. A good run leaves a high that lasts all day. A good race can leave a high that lasts for months."

If she has a bad run, she feels slow and sluggish. "But still I remind myself that it's better than not having run."

She says there are more mental aspects than physical ones that determine whether she feels it has been a great run or a bad one. "Times on specific routes vary by 1 to 2 percent from day to day, but sometimes it just feels so much easier and you feel so much faster even though you're not really. A crap run doesn't ruin your day - it just doesn't elevate it like a good run does. It makes me want to get out there and do a proper job the next time."

She is practical about the training sessions she skips. For her a good mood can be a reason to forgo a run. "Missed runs are missed but leave you more determined to get back out there and enjoy the sense of ease from running on fresh legs. In a happy, relaxed mood, running just doesn't often happen as I am enjoying the moment with whatever else I am doing. Running gives a sense of escape which you need more when you are stressed or unhappy than when you're happy and relaxed."

A run lifts her spirits. "Running in a bad mood is a good way to rid yourself of it. Running when you are stressed or angry is a healthy way to release frustration and leaves you too exhausted to get upset at what was bothering you beforehand."

She always feels better after a run. "Running improves quality of life. It helps with overall health, gives you more energy and helps you to explore your local surroundings which gives you more of a feeling of living in a city rather than just an apartment or a house."

It has improved her health. "Running helps me to keep mild asthma under control, maintain a reasonable level of fitness, and has some spin-offs to mental state of mind, attitude towards life and means you pay more attention to what you eat and drink. I probably need to look more at the last one. I consider myself to be reasonably healthy not just because I run although running helps. Healthy includes attitudes, mental wellbeing, diet, lifestyle balance and not all of these are addressed purely by running."

Becoming a runner has had an impact on her self-esteem and self-image. "I've always been on the underweight side and haven't lost or gained weight since I have been running. But people are less worried about whether I am eating enough as they justify skinniness with doing a reasonable amount of running. It also means that I have such a large appetite that people see me eating more often than before I started running. Being interrogated less often has helped me feel a lot less self-conscious although perhaps this is related to getting older and more accepting of how you are. Also seeing a lot of the good runners being really skinny helps me understand my body type."

She prefers to do her long runs alone and her speed sessions with others. "Speed work I prefer to do in a mixed group as the men have an ability to put on speed that women generally don't have. Women tend to be less aggressive, which counts against us in speed work."

She believes women approach running in a different way than men do. "Pass a woman and they're generally not too bothered – maybe they'll try not to lose too much ground. Pass a man and they'll usually try to pass you back. But they can't. So you end up with some hyperventilating guy slapping around behind you and you slow down so you don't have to call an ambulance. Women tend to be more even pace setters. They pick up distance more easily while men pick up speed more easily."

While she initially took up running because she could do it on her own, she has since found the social aspect of training with others enjoyable. She has made new friends through running. "They're not soul mates but more good acquaintances. You get to know more people to wave at when you cross paths on morning runs, which creates a nice sense of community."

She is considerate when training with others who have less running fitness. "On a few trail runs I've done recently with multi-sport friends who don't do as much running as me, I've hung back and let them set the pace as it was more important to enjoy the day with friends than to go as fast as I could and leave my friends feeling disgruntled and not wanting to invite me back."

She does not follow a training program. "In the lead-up to a marathon or something like that, I'll add some longer runs from about two months out and try to build up to the sort of time I think it would take. I think I do enough on a normal basis to get through an event and that's all I'm really trying to do. I fit in about as much as I can already and don't think I could fit in anything else without significantly impacting on my life."

She hasn't had any injuries from running. "Touch wood - I don't do enough or change my running load suddenly enough."

She does enter running races. "But only to compete against myself and see what time I really can do that distance in. I'm not competitive against others but do strive to push myself against what I think I should be capable of. I don't mind others being better than me but I get annoyed at myself if I am beaten by someone I know I am better than. This is the same for running as for other areas of my life."

She expects to keep running as long as possible – "until I physically can't run anymore."

She has recommended others to start running. "I tell them that I started by running for a few minutes then walking for one minute and gradually building it up to a half-hour jog. I also tell them to run to the next driveway before turning around and see if they can do that in the same time. And I tell them to just try to enjoy being out there and that there will always be someone else slower and someone else faster than them."

CHAPTER 6
Motherhood provides inspiration to run

"Running means freedom, self-expression and an identity other than being a mum: Pat doesn't yell at me [during a tough training session] any less if the kids have been up all night."

Before Becky Pratten had children she was a competitive sports person who ran to keep fit for the team sports she was involved in. She says she ran because she felt she had to, rather than because running was something she really enjoyed. But all that changed when she became a mum.

After she gave birth she initially resumed running to regain fitness – she was no longer able to make the commitment required to be part of a team. Soon, however, Becky discovered that her running became more than just a way to stay fit. She found new meaning in her solitary sport and with it increased motivation and commitment to an activity that had previously felt to be a chore.

By then she had had her second child. She realised that running helped her see herself in other ways – and aided in shaping her identity. "It soon became about having something in my life that was for me and not about the kids. I was a stay-at-home mum and was sick of talking about them," Becky says.

After her third child, she enlisted Pat Carroll as her running coach and joined his running group. And she enjoyed the fact that she was regarded simply as a runner, just like everyone else. "For me running means freedom, self-expression, and an identity other than being a mum. Pat doesn't yell at me [during a tough training session] any less if the kids have been up all night," she says.

While the flexibility of run training makes it easier to fit it into a busy schedule, it is still a challenge for Becky. "Honestly, I find that the toughest bit. I know that it will get easier when the kids can get their own breakfast, but the time commitment for running a marathon is much greater than I can expect to have consistently while the children are small," Becky says.

While Becky has found that setting goals has become more important to her, she has also become more practical about choosing them. "I'm a very outcome-focused person - always setting goals for myself - and babies are not. So to make sure I stay sane I continue making goals for myself but with a difference. I set goals but I am forgiving and what I have found is that it keeps me on task. An example: I ran my first marathon six months after my baby No. 3 was born. I had the goal of completing it. That's a low goal for me, someone who still thinks she'll run a three-hour marathon someday."

Before her first marathon, Becky's longest races had been half marathons. She planned her training and races as usual, she says. When she couldn't stick to her schedule at times, she accepted that was simply a result of being a mum with three kids. Rather than being angry with herself about missing training sessions, she just made sure to do her next session and did not worry about the ones that she had missed. "I know that in goal-setting terms this would be considered a cop-out but for a woman with a new baby it allows a balance and a feeling of control when very little else offers it in new babyhood. And I achieved a goal.

"Being a mother has made me much more relaxed and forgiving of myself and I think has made me a much better runner. I am generally grateful if there is a legitimate reason to miss a few runs, and then I am busting to get back out there when I can."

Her running regime varies. "I check on my husband's support for an upcoming event. If it is going to fit in with us then I will run six days a week for the time leading up to the event. But when the event is over, it becomes more balanced and he is granted much more him-time."

Becky says her husband, parents, siblings and children are all very supportive of her passion for running as they appreciate it is important to her. Even so, "they probably can't quite fully understand just how much it means to me to have it as my own time. I think I have found a balance whereas there may have been a tendency for me to be Mum, and nothing else."

Her running lifestyle has also changed her friends and allowed her to broaden her social horizons. "My old friends probably don't think I'm as much fun because I don't party like I used to: running is my excuse but, honestly, I was bored with their company. Running does provide a fabulous avenue for interacting with people that a 'housewife' would not usually come across," Becky says.

She trains alone as well as with other runners. "I enjoy running with a group. But because I use the time as me-time I need to have some runs when I go it solo or I just do not get that benefit. I have found a girlfriend in the last couple of years who has added a whole new dimension to my running. The social aspect of running is important - and it is not. I'd run without it, but it was something I found to be an unexpected benefit."

She always enjoys her training - sometimes her arrival back home is the toughest part of the workout. "Every run is great. Except when I was still breastfeeding and I would come home and my husband would look frazzled and the other kids would be hungry and screaming, and the enjoyment I got from the run was stripped away instantaneously."

Generally Becky sticks to her training schedule, regardless of her mood which is typically improved after training. "A good long run on the weekend will carry me through to midweek. A speed session will see me through for about 24 hours."
She even enjoys sessions in which she struggles. "I see it as a good training tool for when I feel crap in a race."

At the time of answering these questions, Becky was pregnant with her fourth. She ran until about the 20th week in her previous pregnancy which helped her maintain a good fitness base for when she resumed running after the baby's birth. Placenta previa prevented her from doing the same this time. While she has accepted the fact that she has to take a longer break from running this pregnancy around, it has also increased her motivation to return to training as soon as she can.

"This pregnancy has made me aware that the healthy feeling I get from running can not be found elsewhere. I feel like I can take on the world when I am running consistently. I am mentally more active and on the ball and feel confident I can physically handle most things."

She has found her doctor's attitude towards running positive. "Initially he was very supportive, saying that running while pregnant was great. He did remind me about the Queensland heat though. He also said that the studies he had read said that the baby did not respond well to the presence of lactic acid in the mother, so he advised to seize doing sprint training."

Becky believes runners feel different to non-runners in pregnancy. "Runners are more able to understand the body's responses to certain aspects of the pregnancy. They are probably more likely to listen to their body and respond accordingly. They are probably more comfortable with finding their own limits rather than have them set by some middle-aged male doctor who may never have run a step in his life. The flipside is that I miss the running dearly when I'm pregnant, so there is a little hole currently that a non-runner might not notice."

She recommends taking it easy when resuming run training after giving birth. "I always try to take it slowly. If you are ever going to be forgiving of yourself, immediately after having a baby is when you should.

"Having said that, my philosophy with a new baby is that you are always going to obsess over something, so it may as well be an upcoming event and that will at least take some focus off the new-baby hard work," Becky says.

Running has renewed her enthusiasm for exercise and given her an opportunity to do so when it suits her. "I was a competitive sports person before the children but the commitment needed to be in a team is a major drawback when the family needs to come first. Now that I'm a runner I feel like I'll always be looking for a physical challenge, whereas before I would never say I was committed to sport for life."

CHAPTER 7
Finding the courage to try is all it takes
"I give every training run the respect it deserves and try my hardest."

Cassie Smith, 38, started running in 2004 after she had some health problems. She was also very overweight. "I had a little bit of a health scare so I decided to do the get-fit thing. I started with a personal trainer who I still train with today. I met him after walking the 10-kilometre Bridge to Brisbane in 1 hour and 49 minutes, feeling really unfit and unhealthy, and asked him if he would train me to run," Cassie says.

A lot has changed since then. Cassie is now running regularly and competes in marathons. "Running affects my quality of life more than you could ever imagine. When I don't run for a few days I feel like crap and I guess I need say no more. I have lost almost 30 kilograms so the health benefits are enormous to me."

She swims and cycles as well, which she initially did as cross training for her running but it wasn't long before she entered triathlon races. She is fit, healthy and confident enough to contemplate taking on Ironman - which involves swimming 3.8 kilometres, cycling 180.1 kilometres before running another 42.195 kilometres - and ultarunning. An ultrarun is a race of any distance longer than a marathon. "I am a runner who does triathlons. And the Ironman is set down as a once-only so from there I may just concentrate back on my running again. I wouldn't mind trying a Comrades [annual 89-kilometre road run in South Africa]."

These days her motivation to run is very different. "It has changed big time. I was originally running to lose weight. It has now become such a big part of my life physically, mentally and socially because I just love it so much."

Cassie has been coached by Pat Carroll. "I absolutely follow a training program. Pat has written my programs and I plan my training diary according to the program. I swear by it – and so do most of the people I run with. It does take a lot for me to skip a session. Once my program is mapped out and I am in training for a specific run I will follow it to a tee. Only if I am away with work commitments will I miss a session."

She runs about four times a week, training with Pat Carroll Running Group (PCRG) on Tuesdays and Fridays, as well as with friends on Wednesday and Sundays. "Unless there is a major hiccup I am very consistent. Most of the time running doesn't fit into my life – my life fits into it. I try to give every training run the respect it deserves and try my hardest."

Cassie mixes up her training, enjoying solo sessions as well as those in company. "I must admit I love a good run on my own, particularly if I have had a busy workweek. That's why I love marathon running. I can get out there with my iPod and put the world to rights by running for half a day. In saying that, I would be lost without the group I run with. They are the best bunch of people you could ever meet and I don't know what I would do without them or how I would survive some of the runs we do. When I cross the line of a run I always think of my running buddies and how many hours we have spent together and the support and encouragement they have given me – and, believe me, some days I need lots of it.

She also has found great friends and motivation with PCRG. "Again, what a fantastic bunch of people: the encouragement from these guys is incredible. For me the social aspect of running is very important. The group I run with twice a week and the team at PCRG are such great people. We all seem to have the same objectives in mind and all go through the same thought processes when times get tough."

Chats during training sessions cover a wide range of topics. "We talk about all types of things, from family and work issues to the latest jokes. There is always the discussion of upcoming events and how we are going to motivate each other through the training program."

She keeps track of her runs which helps motivate her to do all her training. "I am onto my third book. It's a *Runner's World* training diary and I swear by it. It does the head in a bit when I see too many dashes in a row, let me tell you."

The people close to Cassie encourage her passion for running. "Absolutely - I have a very supportive husband and family. It can be tough though. When I am in training for an important event, say a marathon which involves pretty much three months of solid training, we don't have much of a social life which can take its toll on the relationship at times. In saying that, he is always there when I cross that line, as are my dad and mum, and my sister and brother-in-law."

She believes it can be hard for others to truly appreciate what running means to a runner. And even the most understanding spouse and family occasionally struggle to cope with the amount of training – and therefore time commitment – of their athlete. "Unless they are a runner other people do not fully understand what running means to you. But I do however think they appreciate its good points and how positively it has changed my life. Again, when it seems like our whole life revolves around running it is easy for loved ones to lose sight of its importance. On our group runs we can often discuss this because it can be something a lot of runners experience."

Her husband and her family think Cassie has changed since she began running. "First and foremost my health and appearance have changed. But I am a much happier and calmer person and definitely much more organised. My priorities in life seem to have changed and they greatly involve most of the people close to me so they love it."

Cassie says her social circle has also altered with her lifestyle. "I have made some fantastic friends [through running] and we seem to understand each other. I haven't actually lost any friends because of running but I certainly have a lot of friends that I either don't see at all or as much because of my running.

"I go to bed much earlier these days, rarely drink and just maintain a different lifestyle all-around," she says.

Cassie loves the way she feels after a great run. "I feel on top of the world. Nothing can take its place really, it is one of the most elevating experiences and it stays with you for days and sometimes weeks and months. A great run can boost me for months. I try to live on these highs for as long as I can."

Like any athlete, Cassie also has days when her body struggles during training or a race. "I just want to forget those ones – they can stay with you for just as long. My last bad run made me very upset for many weeks but it also made me very determined to ensure I did everything possible to avoid it happening again."

Cassie struggled during the 2007 Gold Coast marathon. "I went out too hard which is easy to do. I didn't feel confident going into it and I over-compensated. It is a long 42 kilometres when you feel like shit. I almost pulled out at 26 kilometres but just had to dig deep. I knew if I pulled out that that would be harder to deal with mentally than just having a bad run. I was aiming for a sub-4. I had done all the training and there was no reason why I wouldn't have achieved it. It is so disappointing when you put that much effort in and it fails you. I finished in 4 hours and 28 minutes which is still a great run but I did it really tough."

Rather than wallow in self-pity or feel discouraged, Cassie became more determined in the preparations for her next big event. It paid off with a personal record time. "Knowing that I had the Sydney marathon just three months afterwards I trained like there was no tomorrow. I was so motivated and focused that I did everything right and was determined not to take another run or my training for granted again. I took 26 minutes off my time. Everything went so right – what an unbelievable run."

The factors determining whether she feels it has been a great or a bad run can be both mental and physical. "However, I can tell how I am feeling beforehand which will normally give me a pretty good indication of how I am going to run – which makes me think a lot of it is mental. But, in saying that, it is essential you are very physically prepared at the same time."

Cassie has learnt that fuelling her body properly is essential to her training, especially if she is skipping a few sessions. "If I eat well I train well. If I have missed a few runs and haven't eaten well, it is harder for me to get back into it. But if I have been able to eat well I can't wait to get back out there and pound the pavement."

She always keeps a close eye on her body, trying to nip any potential problems in the bud. "I have been pretty lucky with injuries and try very hard to catch them early if I feel the signs. I did have a lower-back injury after a fall that slowed me down for a few months. It really pulled me up and I seemed to appreciate my running more than ever after that. I was extremely edgy - while my buddies were out there doing a training run I would lay in bed and map out where I thought they would be."

Cassie does her training regardless of her mood, though her frame of mind can affect the quality of her session. "My mood can certainly play a good part in things. If I am in a good mood it can be a great run and it seems easier to get started, but a bad mood can result in me forcing myself to get out there. Afterwards I have never regretted running to pacify a bad mood. It can certainly turn things around for me. When I drive to Southbank [PCRG meeting point] at 5am to start a run - particularly in winter when it is dark - I not only ask myself what I am doing but could never imagine that I would feel as good as I do after the run."

She considers herself to be healthy because she runs. "But, in saying that, I still need to make sure I eat well to keep my weight down so I stay healthy. I never get sick with colds or flus, even training through winter in the freezing cold, so yes I consider myself healthy. I believe that running makes you healthy."

Running has been important to Cassie's self-esteem and self-image. "I am a very different person today than I was before I discovered the pleasure of running. Every aspect of my life has changed because I have a more positive outlook and feel much different about myself. Becoming a runner I can honestly say has changed every single facet of my life - from the people I mix with to the way I feel about myself and my appreciation for both life and small things. Every day is a great day if I have managed a run. Let's just say, once you have run a marathon you can do anything."

Cassie loves racing. "I used to enter everything. If I spotted a 10km or 5km, whatever, I would be in there having a go. Now that I have discovered marathon running I tend to just enter the big ones. I am only really competitive against myself. Although I noticed last week that I was desperately trying to close the gap between me and a runner in front of me during a speed session. I do strive to achieve a better result than the last – I am not really a competitive person by nature but I do work hard."

She recommends running to others and provides practical encouragement. "I have also started some little beginners running groups for my friends to help them. I trained a couple of girls to run the 5km in Bridge to Brisbane and what a buzz to see them finish all smiles. You can't convince people - you can only encourage them."

CHAPTER 8
Being a runner has become a lifestyle

"Running has also taught me never to say never, and that doing something difficult and facing the challenge is so rewarding."

Christina Siu began running in 2005 when she was in her mid 30s. "I was tired of going to the gym, and was inspired by two friends who are runners. They never talked me into running, in fact I've never discussed running with them, but I found their conversations about entering races and about training interesting. I also liked the fact that no fancy equipment is needed, and you can do it anywhere. One of my friends only runs in his lunch hour, as he is busy with his family in the evenings and weekends, so I figured there's really no excuse. At the beginning it was just a give-it-a-go sort of thing. Today, I run because I like running, keeping fit, and it has become a regular part of my life," Christina says.

Becoming a runner has boosted her self-confidence and awareness of her health. "Running helps build my self-esteem as it's something challenging and with consistent effort you can see results. The first time I was able to run non-stop for half an hour I was ecstatic, and that helps you continue on the course and gives you a boost of confidence. I don't remember the details of this particular run, but I think the main impact is the sense of achievement and the rewarding experience you feel when you push yourself just that little bit more."

She surprised herself again when at the age of 40 she began training for the Sydney half marathon, held in May 2008. She enlisted the help of Brisbane-based coach Pat Carroll and completed a long run of 1 hour and 40 minutes in preparation for the race. "At the beginning of the training program I thought I was never going to be able to do that. Every little bit of extra effort you put in, you get something out of. That does great things to your confidence and helps propel you to do more. I've always liked sporty things and the fact that goals are simple and easily measurable. I sometimes wish I could apply my diligence in running to other aspects of life."

Christina runs three to five times a week and is consistent with her training. "Running has now become a regular thing in my life. I even try to fit it in during my holidays," she says. Christina also hikes and does weight training regularly. "I don't have a preference as such because I run to keep fit, challenge myself and to decompress, but I hike to enjoy the outdoors and the scenery. Weight training is just a should-do thing as I find it boring."

The people close to Christina are very supportive of her passion for running. She says they don't all understand what running means to her. "I think my partner does to a certain extent though I don't think others do. However, I don't feel I need to explain to anyone why I run. Running to me means: lone-time, fitness, relaxation, feeling good and being challenged."

A great run leaves her feeling energetic, empowered, happy, and relaxed. Even when her session has been a struggle, she experiences similar emotions. Whether Christina feels it was a great run or a bad one is probably both mental and physical, she says. "Sometimes when you feel tired, or less fit that day, you want to push yourself and you have to win the mind over to do that. If I am not happy with my run, it doesn't ruin my day. It always motivates me to continue because of how good it feels after a run. Bad run or good run, I still feel the runner's high, I still get the benefits and it always improves my day."

She typically feels much better after a run and uses it to lift her spirits if needed. When she skips a few runs because of other commitments or illness, she misses her training and finds it easy to get back into it. "I guess it's because it has become a part of my life now. I feel uneasy and lazy when I don't run. Keeping active is generally very important to me nowadays. Running has improved my life a lot. It's so easy to do - just walk out the door basically - that it is easy to incorporate into any schedule. I feel fitter, healthier and more confident."

She thinks about the health benefits of running and considers herself to be healthy "partly" because of it. "I used to be a smoker. Initially after I quit I couldn't even run for five minutes without feeling chest pains. I hated running back then and never thought I'd be a runner, ever. Today, because I enjoy running so much and enjoy being active in general, I'd never go back to smoking as it is such a conflict."

Christina runs alone. "I don't know if I'd enjoy running in a group as I have never tried. I tend to do things on my own, and am quite happy to do so. But I do think a coach [to run with] would help to improve performance and maintain motivation. I also enjoy the solitude of running on my own with just my iPod on.

"I don't consider myself competitive when I run. I run for myself and myself only. I challenge against myself, and don't really care that much what others are doing. My partner often says that I am hard on myself and am competitive, and I think sometimes I am, but it has to work with my values. I also don't consider myself all that competitive in other areas of my life. I have an internal compass and I follow that."

Christina struggled with an injury when she was not following a specific training program. "I wanted to try for a half marathon about a year ago but realised I was overtraining because I was getting knee pain. I slowed my training down and increased my kilometres slowly. Not being able to run was disappointing, so I stopped for a few weeks and then slowly started running again."

Becoming a runner has changed Christina's life. The rewards she treasures most are the sense of freedom and achievement it has brought her. "It has made me value exercise and being healthy. It has also taught me never to say never, and that doing something difficult and facing the challenge is so rewarding. I expect to keep running until my body can give no more. Being a runner has become a lifestyle."

CHAPTER 9
Running has always made me feel confident
"I love the atmosphere of the events that I compete in; I think the competitive air is really motivating and inspirational."

Davina Alston, now in her late 30s, has been a runner for most of her life. She did short and middle distance running at local and state levels during her school years. "I have run most of my adult life for general fitness mostly. I have taken it more seriously in the past four years with a greater focus on building a solid base for endurance running as well as preparing for events. I participated in athletics as a child as my father was my coach and I followed in the footsteps of my two elder sisters, one of which competed at a national level," Davina says.

As an adult her motivation for running is her desire to stay fit and her association with the sport. "I always remembered feeling really confident when I trained hard as a child; I needed to have some personal goals rather than just a focus on work-orientated goals. I felt that my work was taking over my mind so I needed to set some challenging personal goals."

Davina swims and cycles as cross training. "I prefer running as it is so easy just to strap on the shoes, slap on my watch and hat, and away I go. Running is also an all-year sport."

She typically runs five times per week and usually trains alone. "I work with so many people and am constantly bombarded with phone calls and conversations throughout the day: the 45 to 60 minutes I spend running is my time back. I do run with my husband once or twice a week and that is fine - he doesn't like to talk."

Davina loves to keep track of her training sessions. "I am a bit fanatical with my running diary as I enjoy entering details between bites at breakfast - watch in one hand, calculator and pen in the other. Last year I recorded all my running days and times on a calendar on the fridge. I spent most of the New Year weekend typing it up and setting my goals for this year against it."

She doesn't follow a specific training program and believes her running would benefit if she did. "I must admit I need to improve on this point as although I keep a note of my running achievements and training, they aren't always planned. I think I could be a much better runner if I stuck to a regimented plan."

Davina has to take extra care of her knees to avoid injury. "I get a niggly runner's knee sometimes and it has sadly flared up just recently. I know that it is a result of my pushing up the weekly mileage suddenly so I should learn my lesson.

She has had to take a long break from her run training twice in the past two years, which has been challenging. "I had some surgery on another health issue two years in a row. It is hard to get back into it, as I'm not allowed to do anything physical for six weeks, but it makes me very determined to start as soon as a second over six weeks happens. Becoming a runner has improved my life. I expect to keep running until I can't bend over to lace up my shoes."

Her key driver for running is the satisfaction the sport gives her. "Running a long slow distance is the best to really give me a buzz. Nothing else can beat the feeling of achieving a good distance, especially with some hills dispersed among the kilometres. Although running is an individual sport, you are still competing against yourself and the clock. This also helps me focus."

Her husband is supportive as he is an avid cyclist. "We are both often out on the road so neither one of us feels guilty about not spending extra time with each other. We often head out quite early so we can still spend the full days together on the weekend. Often during the week when I know I have a huge workload I will keep my run for the evenings as it helps me decompress from the day."

Family and colleagues are also encouraging. "I think my sister thinks I'm a bit obsessed but she still supports my drive and commitment to my running. My colleagues at work are impressed and I think my determination is starting to rub off on a few people who have mentioned they've started running."

Not everyone may understand what it takes to train with the aim of improving her best times. "Many of my friends and family think I run to stay healthy and are not aware of the preparation and training I do to make the most of my running."

Most people seem to first notice her physique, rather than her attitude. "Often people comment on how I look more than how I am in myself – although I've always been slim I've become leaner especially when I'm putting in the long kilometres."

Davina loves her long runs. "Believe it or not, the best I feel is when I've run more than 10 kilometres and in particular the half marathon is my favourite. I often have a bit of an out-of-body experience as I know my feet start to hurt and my head is hot, but I feel like I could become Forrest Gump and keep on running."

A great run leaves her with a feeling of mental elation. "When I look back in my log book at those times the comments are usually `Felt free' or `Focused'. I can definitely have a much better day when I've had a positive run. I feel like I've kicked a personal goal and nothing can bring me down."

Like any runner, Davina also has days when her body is not cooperating during a training session. "I feel like my feet are made of cement. I mostly have a rotten run when I'm heading into my period or I am just plain tired from the week. It upsets me a bit to think that work especially gets into my head too much and then interferes with my concentration or personal running time. A bad run is a combination of both physical factors, such as cement feet, and mental factors, such as lack of concentration," Davina says.

A run that was a struggle is never a reason to give it up. "I've never felt like not putting back on the shoes again after a bad run. I just keep on going. I am still pleased that I have been out on the road. I think I would feel more off if I didn't go out and still felt down."

She rarely skips a training session and is creative about making the time in her busy schedule. "I absolutely hate missing my runs because of other commitments especially work. I make it my business to squeeze a run in after work, even if it is a short one. There is travel involved in my work, but I always make time to pack the shoes and find a path to run on. Many of my trips are to capital cities so I can check out the sights. I bought a great book recently about running tracks in Australia so now I am more motivated than ever to run while travelling. My husband and I travelled to the United States recently and the highlight of our trip was to run through and around Central Park and New York. If I know that my travel time is when I would normally run, early morning or late in the evening, I sometimes plan my rest day to fall on these days."

A bad mood is certainly never a reason to skip a run. "I run no matter the mood. I did an amazing run once when I had a terrible argument with someone and I swear I felt like running and never stopping. I think it helped me as it gave me my time back again."

She always feels better after a run than she did before. "Even though I love to run I can still wake up some mornings and think how much I'd like to sleep in but once I'm back from my run, either good or bad, I'm pleased I did it."

Overall becoming a more consistent and purposeful runner has improved the quality of her family life, she says. "My husband and I both enjoy our physical activity so much and find we talk about our achievements and plans for the next ones like other people talk about their night out to the pub. We have met some great like-minded people through our events especially the triathlons that we do together as a team."

Being a runner is definitely a lifestyle, Davina says. "My husband and I love our sport and would choose that over most other social activities. We recently went away to Noosa for a week's holiday and swam and ran as if we were at training camp. As sad as this sounds we both felt so great afterwards as we were able to relax around the sport we did, rather than having to go to work."

She appreciates the health benefits that come with being a runner and considers herself healthy because she exercises regularly. "I find the articles and books that I read very interesting when I learn more about the implications and benefits of running. I feel sorry for people who don't exercise - not necessarily run - as they are missing out on such a great feeling about themselves."

Her running lifestyle has also helped her in her career. "I have a job which requires me to be a figure head in my organisation so it is important that my running helps me represent a positive and healthy image. Running also gives me more confidence to carry out my role which is a management role largely dependent on strong leadership skills. I know that a personal achievement of a marathon or hill running also helps deliver this. Often it is more about if I can do this – a half marathon or something similar - well I can do anything. The other part of it is driven by the fact that I look better and feel better in me as a result, which also allows for a more confident nature. Let's face it women can be a bit vain."

She enjoys racing. "I love the atmosphere of the events that I compete in. The competitive air is really motivating and inspirational. I love to compete and prove to myself I am successful at something. That doesn't necessarily mean I need to win but I need to prove a point. This is the same feeling I get from my studies and work life. I have achieved some great milestones in my life so it isn't a new habit."

She celebrates such accomplishments in her running by rewarding herself. "Sadly yes, much to my credit card's dismay. I ran the Sydney City to Surf last year for the first time with a really good personal time, which will put me up in the red group this year. So I headed into Castlereagh Street to treat myself to a piece of jewellery," Davina says.

Davina believes that women approach their running differently than men do. "We are more competitive than men. I noticed the competitiveness of women first when I used to play team sports at school including netball and hockey. It frightened me to say the least sometimes that playing a team sport with women is bad for your health. Maybe women's competitiveness has been driven by the fact that historically women had to play the submissive role, but as our role in society has become more dominant and we have more opportunities it rubs off into our actions, sport and work. I think Paul Radcliffe is a great example of a very competitive woman and also Emma Snowsill. A woman's competitiveness is more focused and determined."

CHAPTER 10
Taking charge of your destiny
"I realised there were two options left to me; I could continue to get old or I could do something about it."

Diane Soffe had always been active and played netball competitively. But with the arrival of children and moving home both within her native New Zealand and overseas, sports had taken a backseat. Their first child was born in 1980. Diane's young family moved to an isolated rural area near Taranaki, New Zealand. Then the family moved to Singapore for three years where Diane played netball again and ran occasionally with the Hash House Harriers. While her level of activity wasn't anything like it had been previously, she still considered herself to be in good shape.

In fact Diane's fitness had dropped significantly which she realised when she moved back to the town she had grown up in. It was 1999 and Diane was 42. "Some of my old netball buddies caught up with me and asked me to play in a Masters netball team and travel with them to the New Zealand Masters games. It sounded like a great idea – I loved the girls and couldn't wait to get back into it," Diane says.

Unfortunately, that proved harder than she had expected. "I went to the first practice and it was all downhill from there. The others had never really stopped playing competitively and I thought I'd just step right back in there and take up where I left off."

Having played netball for so many years, Diane's mind still knew exactly what to do. But by neglecting her fitness, Diane's body wasn't able to cooperate. "My mind could see the gaps but do you think I could get to them? The legs just no longer had the ability. I went home very chastened and feeling rather foolish. I then had to spend the next week or two trying to come up with some excuse so that I didn't have to go to the Masters games with the team. It turned out that I didn't even have to invent a story – I had done such damage to my Achilles tendons that no amount of mind-over-matter was going to do the job anyway."

Diane was shocked. The realisation she no longer was the sporty and fit person she always had been - and still had considered herself to be – was tough to deal with. "As I lay on the couch knowing that all my old mates - who were just as old as I was - were away being active and having a great time, I realised there were two options left to me; I could continue to get old, or I could do something about it."

Diane decided to start walking five days a week as soon as her Achilles injury had healed. She also resolved to improve her nutrition, and asked a dietician for advice. The dietician told Diane to make a few simple changes: more vegetables, grains and lean meat. "I wasn't overweight, just a tad flabby. But I'd been having problems with skin conditions, allergies and general unwell-ness. The netball fiasco just brought it all to a head and was really the point where I had to make some conscious decisions," says Diane.

Diane eventually began walking daily. As she got fitter, she introduced short stretches of running during her walks, such as from one power pole to the next. "That was the beginning of my love for running." Like many people who start running and feel their fitness improving, Diane thought doing more was better. "I found a nice block to run around and set about getting faster every time I ran it. When I was getting out there six nights a week, you can imagine what happened to the body – a slight case of burnout. In my ignorance I thought that you just tried to get faster and faster. It sounded fine to me."

Diane realised she needed advice and company for her training. An ad in the local newspaper that the Hawera Harriers had an open day for new runners the following Saturday caught her eye. "I took the bull by the horns, as every good New Zealander knows how to do, and turned up. This was my next major learning curve. Not a lot of women belong to our local club. In fact only one other woman was among the gathering of about 15 that day. Here I was, not a clue what I was in for, surrounded by all these men who looked very professional in their club shirts,

Asics shoes and their muscled legs. There was no backing out now. To my great relief I had a fantastic day. We had a wonderful pack-run around our beautiful rural cross-country course, which I came to know very well over the next several years. The guys were just wonderful, so encouraging, and the other woman was very pleased to have some female company."

After that first run with the Hawera Harriers, Diane was invited to participate at a neighbouring club's event the next Saturday. Reluctantly and intimidated, she agreed. "On arrival I was met with a picture of very professional-looking athletes all warming up and looking very serious. I was given a club shirt. I took so long in the change room that I nearly missed the start of my race – I thought that I wasn't good enough for all this running-shirt stuff. I felt so embarrassed heading out the door, wondering how on earth I'd ever got myself into such a position. Fortunately, the start was moments away – no warming up for me and no time to back out. I just wanted it over and done with. The gun went off and I experienced my first closed-handicap cross-country race. I loved it. I wasn't as fast as some, but neither was I as slow as others. These were just ordinary people after all."

Ordinary and yet amazing – Diane found that running was a great way to meet people who cemented her motivation. "I met a very inspirational lady that day. She was in her 60s and had run marathons all over the world. She wasn't particularly wealthy and not very fast either, but she had enjoyed so many wonderful times away. Within the year of meeting her, this lovely lady suffered a major brain tumour from which she never fully recovered. She'd often come to watch us run in the following years and was always as encouraging as she'd been that first day I met her. I'm still grateful to her for showing me that even beginning as a Masters runner, there was so much to try to achieve and enjoy."

Diane's introduction to group running and races was a positive experience, allowing her to make new friends and find other ways to enjoy her running. "We were small in numbers, so we were all encouraged to take part in all inter-club activities. Many other clubs would have two meets each Saturday: one for the competitive runners and another for the social runners. I'm so pleased our club didn't do that, as I may never have got out there and really seen what I could do and the fun I could have by competing, even at this late stage.

"The feeling of camaraderie, the chat about what we'd done, and the talk about our times and what we'd do next week was such fun on the way home. I knew it was time to buy my club shirt and become part of this unassuming, committed group of weekend warriors. That was the beginning of a wonderful association I had with a very special group of rural town New Zealand people. I learned so much from that bunch over the years. They were never too busy or grand to help anyone who wanted to ask as many questions as I seemed to find."

The club consisted of a wide variety of athletes. "We had an elite runner who ran for New Zealand at the international Mountain Running Championships. Our oldest runner was in his 70s, and we had some children who came every week too – one of them is now on a running scholarship at an American university. We all mixed in. No one was ever left behind. Everyone was always pleased for the success of others, whether that was reflected glory from our elite runner or a new runner completing their first lap of the cross-country course. It really made what can be a very solitary sport a wonderfully companionable one."

Diane quickly developed a passion for competitive running. She enlisted a coach with two friends, Christine and Sandy who had also joined the Hawera Harriers. The three women in their 40s ran up to 130 kilometres a week. "We still laugh about it when the three of us get together. Christine and Sandy blame me for all the blisters and sore muscles, but I know they loved it really. We spent hours together on the road, sorting out all sorts of problems for each other. The companionship was very special and has created a bond that we'll always share, even now that we live miles apart. Every now and then I just had to pinch myself to realise I was having such a good time doing something that I really didn't even know existed."

A few years later Diane moved again and she now lives in West Papua where she does most of her running alone, often on a treadmill. Health and fitness are still major motivators but she has found others too. "I realise that to keep my body healthy, I need to stay active. It's about 10 years since I realised how unfit I'd let myself get and I don't want to feel that again. However, over the years I've come to love the challenge of pitting myself against my ability to stay competitive and to keep running. Because I live in this isolated place now, I've had to substitute running with my mates with a desire to stay fit enough to be able to compete when we eventually go back to New Zealand."

Diane says that running in West Papua is both her biggest saviour and her biggest frustration. "It's my saviour because it's something I can do in this very remote mining camp. I work long hours as a teacher at the expatriate school here. We live in a very small community, 6000 feet (1829 metres) up a mountain, so it's important to be able to get out and do something. Options are a bit limited. I've learned that it certainly helps my state of mind to run regularly, so I'm not about to give it up.

"It's frustrating because there are only two outside choices of where to run: up or down the mountain. We're also very confined within our small housing area. We have a good gym and I have a love/hate relationship with the treadmills there. I'd never run on one before we came here and I hope to never run on one after we leave. Give me the great outdoors anytime. It also rains nearly every afternoon so I do most of my runs in the afternoon in the pouring rain. We do have a very second-rate artificial turf track which is only 300 metres and has concrete under the matting. I know exactly how many circuits equate to exactly how many miles. I've devised some very unique and odd ways of keeping track of how many laps I've done. I usually have to share it with large numbers of Indonesian soccer players. They are finally getting used to me but it's interesting trying to dodge balls and big men running fast. At least it staves off boredom, as I have to keep my wits about me."

While grateful that she can keep up her training in West Papua, she wishes she had other people to run with and local races to enter. "I also really miss my running club mates, and just having people to talk to about all those dumb things that runners talk about – aches and pains, programs, weight, upcoming events, change in weather. No other women run seriously here and the few men who do are often on shift work so can never be relied on as running buddies. I miss having events to look forward to too, whether they are competitive or just fun. My goal is to treat myself to some marathons - I've only run halve marathons so far - around the world once we are finished here."

To concentrate her training, Diane enlisted the help of Pat Carroll who wrote a training program for her which has her running five days a week. Diane used to aim for six days a week but found it hard to sustain. "I love the program. It has given me real focus. It's varied enough to be enjoyable and is very challenging. Having the two days off has given a little more flexibility too."

Diane's husband and kids, the latter now adults, encourage her running. "My husband is fantastic. He doesn't run but he's very supportive of me. He also knows how much better I am when I'm running so is happy to encourage me out there. He says I'm a much easier person to live with when I'm running regularly. He's also the first to ask if I need a run if I'm getting a bit disagreeable. We have three kids in their 20s. I remember driving off to a Saturday fixture all on my own one day and working out that we'd taken kids to Saturday sport for 25 years. Now it was my turn. The kids think it's great that I still run. Our 27-year-old son took it up last year and the two of us did several trail runs when we were back in New Zealand at Christmas time. He thought it was great that he could go running with his mother. I wasn't so sure, when I followed him down the trail at a greater distance than I care to admit to – 27 and I was still 'running after him'. I do know the kids are pretty proud of what I still do with my running."

Diane says becoming a runner has changed her, as she found a connection with running that goes beyond health and fitness. "I am quite staggered at the hours I've invested in it over the last 10 years. I really can't imagine my life without it. I love the feeling of inner confidence it gives me just to know I can push my body in this way. It's not a comparison thing with anyone else, or a better-than-you feel. It's just a personal challenge and sense of achievement every time I go out there. Being a runner is a lifestyle for me. It really underpins my life. It's a constant challenge and interest."

Diane is proud of her accomplishments and, like most runners, she's modest about them. When considering the comments she made for this book, she said, "I'm a bit embarrassed, as it sounds as though I might be quite a good runner, and that's not the case at all. I just love the challenge and the doing of it. I love trying to improve – for what? Well, goodness knows."

CHAPTER 11
Running is my passion
"A great run feels like the hard work is getting easier."

Fiona Paul began running in mid-2004 after she watched a friend compete in a triathlon. She had previously been a swimmer but hadn't exercised for about five years. "I thought it looked fun. I wanted to be able to do a triathlon, only I couldn't run at all. My first run was on a treadmill and I ran one-and-a-half kilometres. My calves ached for two days after," Fiona says.

Even so, Fiona persisted with her run training which paid off. Then she wanted more. "Once I began to be able to run around the local block once, something in my brain kicked in and all of a sudden I wanted to be able to run the block twice, then three times. I found running more addictive and it did become interesting to me to see how far I could run. It was very challenging and rewarding to be able to run a little bit further each time."

Now the 24-year-old lists running as her core passion. "It's my thing and something that I feel I can do well – through my own expectations of myself. I tried many different sports and activities when I was in school and university. I tried gymnastics, hockey, netball, singing, playing the saxophone and finally found my niche with running. I was never passionate about these other activities, nor did I feel it really was a part of me. Running is where I feel comfortable and by running I am becoming who I want to be. I have a sense of accomplishment and I can add value from the knowledge I collect."

One of her favourite quotes is by the late Dr George Sheehan who wrote great books about running including *Running & Being: The Total Experience*.

"The more I run, the more I want to run, and the more I live a life conditioned and influenced and fashioned by my running. And the more I run, the more certain I am that I am heading for my real goal: to become the person I am."

Fiona runs four days a week. She does her training sessions after work which is always a challenge. Her alternative is to train before work which means getting up at 4:30am. "I just can't wake up at that time, so I go in the evening. Sometimes things come up and I might reshuffle my days but overall I'm quite consistent. I live an hour from the city and work, a full-time job. I run after work three days a week and then usually get home about 8:30pm. I have tried many times to run in the morning but I struggle way too much. The only way I can run in the morning is if I catch an early train to work and then run from there with a friend. Knowing that I have committed to run with someone else or a race are the only things that get me out of bed to run in the morning."

Melbourne-based Fiona enlisted the help of Brisbane-based running coach Pat Carroll who now devises training programs for her. "I signed up to online training to improve my times and give myself some consistency. I have the motivation to go for a run, but I never knew exactly what to run and I would either end up procrastinating or running an easy session. I was not pushing myself. The programs that Pat has given me are perfect for me. The programs are designed for my ability and goal times are challenging but achievable. With online training, I like being able to report back on sessions. It keeps the motivation levels high. It's always great to report back on achieved goal times. And having a program means you are able to psych yourself up for what's coming."

She turns to Pat via email with any running-related questions. "We've never met but he knows my running better than I do. He is someone I definitely respect and has so much knowledge on the sport. The information that he gives me I don't query whatsoever. What he says goes."

She keeps track of her training in a spreadsheet and lists details such as how she felt during the session, as well as the distance she ran and details about her heart rate. Fiona does skip training sessions on occasion and feels guilty for doing so unless it was illness that prevented her from running. When she skips a few sessions in a row, she can find it hard to get back into the training routine. "I definitely miss it. I feel like I'm wasting away. If I'm sick I accept it more. If it's a case of just being busy, I get frustrated that I'm not getting time to do something for me. Generally I would say it's harder to get back into it but it is dependent on how long I've had off and what goals I have. I went away for three weeks last year and it was about four weeks before I could really get back into it. Before my travels I was training for the Great Ocean Road half marathon. After my travels I didn't have a goal that I was passionate about to train for. Just recently I missed a week of training purely because I was busy. I stressed during the week that I was losing fitness but I found it easy to get back into it the following week. If anything, I felt better."

Fiona loves racing and regularly does, for several reasons. "Entering a race gives me motivation to train. Often I run races where the course is not normally open to foot traffic so it's quite a good experience. I love driving around Melbourne and thinking, 'I've run over this bridge or through this tunnel and on this road'. Racing is also when I truly feel part of a wonderful community of people."

She is competitive when she runs. "I've not placed anywhere near the top 3 of a race and I don't expect to. On average I place roughly in the top 10 percent to 12 percent of races for my category, nothing special to most people but I am stoked about it. When I see the results of the race it does drive me to train harder to see if I can improve further. My biggest competition is the clock. I ran in Run for the Kids in Melbourne. There were thousands of people running in front me. I was purely in the pack and all I thought was, 'This is about me versus the clock'."

She says she is less competitive in other areas of her life. "I don't have the tunnel vision of determination that I get with running. Because of my running I aim to be the best I can be in other areas of my life but I don't necessarily have the same passion about it. Running is different because other areas of my life are shared: family, friends, work. Running, however, is something I've chosen for me."

Her life and lifestyle have changed since she became a runner. "We all choose different priorities and lifestyles. When I was 18, my priority on a Friday night was to consume as much alcohol as possible by 10:30pm and head for a dance floor. Now my priority on a Friday night is to consume as much pasta as I can and head to bed by 10:30pm in preparation for my long run on Saturday morning."

A few of Fiona's friends are intrigued and encouraging of her running while others resent her commitment to the sport because it means she has less time to spend with them. "Some friends are very supportive and frequently ask how my running is going and wish me luck for races. Other friends think I'm wasting time and don't understand that I might like to go to bed early on a Saturday night if I'm running a race Sunday morning."

She says that some friends do not appreciate what running means to her. "Some completely understand – admittedly they are also involved with sports - but some definitely don't understand. I have good friends and family who simply think my running is an inconvenience to life, i.e. if I can't go out because of a race. It does get upsetting because I don't race all the time and when I do it truly means something to me. I'm not sure some people understand that running is a big part of who I am. The people that understand it see that I have become more confident within myself, which I believe is true. I'm happier in myself."

Fiona has made new friends through running and hasn't lost touch with her non-running friends. "They might not all understand the need-to-run part of me but they are still really great friends."

Fiona believes that running is important to her self-esteem. "I feel great internally and externally. I am happy with my running achievements and my self-esteem is high when I have a good session and I reach goals and targets. Being part of the running community also boosts self-esteem, as I am surrounded by people who encourage and respect me for running. My body has never been in better shape and I'm happy with how I look. I feel great for having a fit body but it's not the reason I train hard nor is self-image in my mind when I'm pushing myself to get to the top of a hill. That's just the passion to run it in a faster time than the previous session. When my body started to become more toned from running, in my mind these forming muscles meant my body wanted to run. It was ready for it. It was a good turning point to see my body change in terms of what I felt I could do."

During some training sessions and races those changes are evident. "A great run feels like the hard work is getting easier. It feels like I've reached another stepping stone towards a goal. I feel more confident and think that perhaps I am a good runner."

On days when running seems a struggle Fiona wonders why she bothers. "Why am I busting my guts when all I'm doing is hurting? I also feel frustrated and think I can't do this anymore."

She believes often the reason for a poor session is a mental one. "There are times my brain is not engaged with my body. If I have to talk myself into going for a run, I know deep down that I'm not enthused and I know that I will stop a few kilometres into it. If I stop once I will then keep stopping every few 100 metres if I continue. There are of course physical boundaries, i.e. injuries, but they are easier to deal with because of the physical pain when running. When it's a mental battle I think I can't do it today but I'm not really sure why I can't do it. Sometimes – just because. The good thing is that the subconscious thought can work the other way. Yesterday it looked like it was going to rain just as I was about to go out for a time-trial run. Part of my brain was trying to talk my body out of going for a run. But I knew I had the motivation to go because last time I did this time trial I did poorly and I now had the chance to conquer it. And I did."

A great run will boost her spirits for at least a day. When Fiona has a fantastic race, she will enjoy her runner's high for a week. "The races are where my hard training is expressed. So if I do well I celebrate it. Following a race, friends may ask how I went and when I tell them I feel a recreation of the excitement and it boosts my mood again. If I'm not happy with a run I will feel a bit low for a few hours but I tell myself the next session will be OK and I go into it thinking that. If the second session is a bad one, I might be inclined to skip the third session, have a mental break and be prepared again for the fourth."

Fiona is more likely to run when she is in a good mood than in a bad one. "Sometimes a run is the best recipe to turn a bad mood around. My mind is cleared and I feel happy that I'm doing something for myself. I also feel a sense of achievement."

Leading an active lifestyle has many benefits. "I feel I have a great quality of life. I achieve more out of my day and make the most of time. I believe if I am active and positive with my fitness, then my lifestyle and my attitude to everyday tasks will also be active and positive. My mind is clear after a run and I am able to think about my direction for many things in my life. Running balances me. I figure if I can work hard for a run, I can work hard for other tasks or goals, and vice versa."

She regards running as very important to her health. "I was so shocked at how unfit I was when I first started running. I probably don't really think about the health benefits in detail, only that being fit is important to me and by being healthy I feel good."

She doesn't consider herself to be healthy simply because she runs. "To be healthy I think the human body has other requirements, such as diet and sleep. I eat fairly well but I still think I can improve my health through my diet. I also think sleep and rest are vital to being healthy. Whilst I love running, if I kept running without a rest I would wear myself down pretty quickly. I need to rest and have enough sleep in order to become stronger and fitter."

Fiona likes running solo as well as with others. "Every week I like to do two sessions by myself. It's the best me-time I can get. I can really tune into myself. It's almost like a present to me. Sometimes I run with one or two friends during the week and they are great with encouraging and helping me. They are faster than me, so they have the ability to talk to me at my pace. I run with a mixed group on a Saturday morning and I truly look forward to it. The group is such a wonderful bunch of people. We might go for a two-hour run which I dread if I have to do it on my own. We all run together and it makes those long distances so much easier. I have no preference for running with women or mixed groups."

Fiona enjoys socialising with other runners and the motivation she gets from doing so. "The most important social aspect is to be surrounded by like-minded people. Runners understand runners and meeting each other is a great chance to talk and share our week's running sessions, races, times and injuries. Runners can constantly add value to each other. I run my weekly sessions at a track that is a popular spot for runners. When I am by myself, I will run past a group or pair of runners and catch part of their sentences to each other. More often than not, they are talking about a previous race or session. The tone of the runners is positive and upbeat. I find it really uplifting."

Fiona likes to chat with the other runners during sessions if possible. Topics can be light-hearted and serious. They can be very engaging. Her Saturday group often splits up according to the distance they plan to run. Often the groups will run the first part together. "One Saturday I ran with the 7km group. We ran with the 15km group for about 3km before separating. Whilst both groups were merged at the start I began talking to another runner I hadn't met before. We spoke about running, work, holidays and before I knew it I ran 15km when my intentions were to run 7km."

During another session Fiona was running alone along her usual route in her neighbourhood. The final 1km of that route is straight. "I always feel like stopping there. On this particular day, half-way along that 1km stretch, a lady sat in a wheelchair in the front of the aged-care home watching me run by. I kept plodding along. As I was about to run past her I saw that she was saying something to me. I had my earphones in so I missed what she said. I stopped to take my earphones out. I expected she was going to ask me what the time was. I said, 'I'm sorry, what did you say?' and she repeated what she had said, 'You're doing a really good job.' It made me think how lucky I am to have the ability to run. If I miss a day's running, at worst I might lose a tad of fitness but at least I can go out tomorrow and go for a run. Whenever I'm tired and people say that I might be overdoing it and that the body isn't meant to take so much pounding of the pavement, I just think that I was given a healthy set of lungs and two legs so I'm going to use them."

In March 2006 Fiona had an experience she still regards as the worst in her running career so far. She followed a route that had taken her further from home than usual. "I began to feel sudden bowel movement and was not near any toilets whatsoever. It was an awful experience and I couldn't hold on until I got home. I guess in one way I was lucky – I was wearing tight shorts. I walked home, showered of course and threw the clothes that I was wearing in the bin. I lay on the couch feeling miserable and embarrassed, although no one saw me. I couldn't understand why something I loved would do that to me. I flicked on the TV just in time to see the last part of the women's marathon in the Commonwealth Games: Kerryn McCann winning the gold medal in such an unforgettable finish. Seeing that race kept the running flame alive in me, though I still didn't run for a good couple of weeks."

For Fiona the single-most important thing about running is her drive. "Having a passion for running means I will continue to put in my best effort. When I feel low from a bad session, it's the passion that drives me to put on the running shoes again. When I achieve a goal, it's because of the passion that I am immensely happy about it. As above, there are many influences as to why running is valuable but I do believe there's a core central where it all stems from and, for me, the core central is definitely the passion."

CHAPTER 12
Forging lifelong bonds along the trails

"Running has brought me lots of good adventures, challenges and new friendships."

Fiona Skinner has been a runner for more than a decade. This extremely modest 34-year-old has since completed five 100-kilometre Oxfam Trailwalker events, a mostly off-road foot race that raises money for charity. Her fastest Trailwalker finish is a swift 17 hours. She has raced the challenging 45-kilometre off-road Six Foot Track trail run four times and has finished two Ironman triathlons.

Fiona began running in 1997 because she wanted to shed a few pounds. The Australian was living in Japan at the time and had added 10 kilograms to her regular 55-kilogram frame in less than six months. Since then she has found many other reasons than weight management to stick to her running regime. "I continue run to keep my weight down but also have found running to provide a mental clarity and health as well as a feeling of happiness and satisfaction in achievement," Fiona says.

Her passion for running was not love at first sight but developed over time. "I was never overly partial to running and tended to prefer swimming, bushwalking and cycling. However in the past three years running has brought me lots of good adventures, challenges and new friendships. This has in turn meant that an activity that was during Ironman training about five years ago a huge chore and struggle has become one I look forward to three to four times a week."

Fiona will often organise to do her running with friends and trains regularly with a group led by running coach Tim Lindop. All the benefits of running consistently have motivated her to fit it into a busy lifestyle. "Running means to me a chance to forget about daily work stresses, life stresses, anxiety and an opportunity to switch off, relax with friends and enjoy nature. Running fits into my life and routine naturally now. I make it a part of my work/life balance and really enjoy the Tuesday and Thursday sessions in Centennial Park with a small running group.

I even feel guilty if I miss it. I enjoy running with my partner and doing my regular weekend long runs with a variety of friends. I find I push myself harder when running with others than alone – I'm less apt to walk if I'm running with others."

The social aspect of running is important to Fiona. "It makes it more fun and I have established a number of good friendships due to the initial running base as their foundation. At times we talk during running, depending on who is in the group and how fast the pace is."

Fiona says that she aims to maintain a steady pace when she is running with other people. She knows her own pace and will stick to it. "If someone is too quick, I let them go for it alone. If someone's lagging I do my best to encourage, cajole and motivate them to continue along."

Like every runner, Fiona feels fantastic during some runs and less energetic during others. "When it's a great run I feel enthusiastic, positive, full of energy – inspired to keep on going and trying to push the envelope. A great run leaves me on a high for a day or so. When it's not, I think better luck next time. I don't tend to get upset if I have a bad run, I just figure that I haven't put in sufficient training, or that my mind or body is tired and isn't up to performing," she says.

Fiona says running always makes her feel better and can cheer her up if she is in a bad mood before her training. She values the health benefits that come with her fitness. "Running is important to my health for weight control and mental happiness – my overall health and wellbeing. Running is important to my self-esteem and self-image. Weight control affects my self-image. I always feel in better shape when I'm running regularly."

Fiona doesn't follow a training program. "My running is more a stress and health outlet, something to do to work up a sweat and get the blood pumping. I like to do it regularly but in recent years I haven't tended to follow a set program. I don't really feel guilty for skipping sessions but I certainly miss them when I do and don't seem to have the same energy levels and drive if I haven't run that day. If I miss a run, I find it hard to get my rhythm back after a break of longer than three days."

She competes in races regularly and, as mentioned, has some impressive finishes to her name. "I don't consider myself competitive in my running against others but I do like to try and beat my PBs in some races. My tendency, though, is to race for the fun and social aspect so I am not overly fussed with my time for most events."

Fiona credits her lifestyle as a runner for many positive experiences. "The majority of my female friends in Sydney I have made through running or triathlon connections. Becoming a runner has opened me up to physical exercise, allowed me to make new friends in a relaxed and fun environment, enabled me to see different parts of the world and some great scenery on my bush runs, relaxed me or given me a healthy stress outlet and helped me maintain a better life balance. I like to think I'll keep running into my 70s."

Fiona cherishes her first marathon which she ran in the same year that she took up the sport. "My best memory involving running was the 1997 Fukuoka marathon where I crossed the finish line in 4 hours and 45 minutes. It was my first-ever long distance race and it really got me into running. The best and most important things about running are the friendships it has brought me and the exhilaration after a good, hard run."

CHAPTER 13
Determined to run again even when they told me I wouldn't

"I feel very free when I run. I love the endorphin rushes and I think a lot - lots of new ideas come to me when I run."

Gina Unwin was a sporty kid who competed in all the races at the athletics carnivals, did Little Athletics and participated in cross-country running carnivals. She loved cross country, the walk, the 1500m and hurdles. Her mother was improving her own fitness and inspired Gina to begin running regularly at the age of 13. They had recently moved to Pymble, NSW, and had a German shepherd named Ash. "My mum was just entering her fitness-freak era and would take Ash running around Pymble and the surrounding suburbs. Mum taught me to run. She taught me technique and how to run up long steep hills, which you had to tackle when you headed out for a run from our house. This was good training as I still enjoy running hills," Gina says.

The teenager ran up to four times a week. Her longest weekly run was 15 kilometres. If she chose company for her runs, it was their dog Ash. "I always ran by myself. I wasn't interested in running with other people, I just never really thought about it. I always ran with music on my Sony Walkman."

In 1995 Gina, by then 19 years old, did her first race with her mum, a 10km that finished in a stadium at Homebush Bay, the site of the Sydney 2000 Olympics. Gina ran 49 minutes and 49 seconds. It is still one of her best running memories. "My first race with my Mum always has a special spot as well as my first half marathon with her," Gina says.

Mother and daughter have done 10 races together. They established a tradition of celebrating afterwards with fish and chips accompanied by a glass of wine in Manly. Unfortunately Gina's body started protesting after she did her first half marathon. What later turned out to be an iliotibial band (ITB) problem cut short her training, before soon stopping her from running altogether. "I could run about 20 minutes and then suffered intense pain. It came on so fast that I just couldn't run."

It was the beginning of a painful and frustrating five-year period with endless visits to doctors, physiotherapists and other experts including an osteopath. "I was devastated during that time. I remember seeing a lot of doctors, crying every time they disappointed me with no solutions. One orthopedic surgeon told me that I might have to get used to the idea that I'd never run again. I committed to Pilates three times a week for two years to try to fix it. I was determined that I would run again."

While Pilates helped strengthen her body and improved her posture, she still couldn't run without pain. In 2002 someone she met at a party told her that surgical release of an ITB was not only a possibility but also highly successful. She was given the name of a specialist, Dr Ken Creighton, and made an appointment to see him. Entering his office provided her with renewed hope. "I hadn't seen anyone who was an athlete specialist. All over his office are framed sporting memorabilia, signed by rugby players, skiers, runners, you name it. There were 10 to 15 sports on his office walls. All these photos were signed by the athletes. They had written things like, 'Thanks Ken you gave me my career back', and 'I'd never be No. 1 in the world without you'. I remember looking around this room and thinking, 'Finally I am in the right place'," Gina says.

Dr Creighton recommended Gina undergo a surgical procedure to release her left ITB that had stopped her from running for so long. She went to the hospital two weeks later to have it done. "I was in and out in a day. My sister picked me up. Six weeks later I could literally run as long as I wanted."

With her newfound freedom to resume running, Gina was able to think about athletic goals again and found one soon. By mid-2003 she decided to train for Ironman Australia. However, this time her right ITB started protesting and she had that side surgically released in December 2003. She was soon able to return to training and finished Ironman Australia five months later – swimming 3.8 kilometres, cycling 180.1 kilometres and running 42.195 kilometres. She sent her finisher photo not only to Dr Creighton but also to the orthopedic surgeon who had told her she'd never run again.

Her worst running experience is the time it took to find someone who appreciated the importance of fixing her injury. "Not being able to run for five years because of ITB, and the lack of understanding of the requirement to fix the problem really pissed me off for a long time."

Gina has completed numerous running races and triathlons, as well as the Sydney Oxfam Trailwalker 100km off-road footrace and the six-day 600km Mark Webber Challenge adventure race. In Ironman an athlete typically spends half the time in the race cycling, a sport Gina prefers to running in some ways. "The only reason I love cycling more is because I am better at it. I feel at one with my bike when I ride it and I love the speed as well. I do just love being on my bike. It is different to running though, as when I cycle I don't think laterally as much and I don't get so many endorphin rushes. Together running and cycling probably feed slightly different emotional and physical needs but together they pretty much tick all my boxes. Adventure racing is a lot more complex and I love it for different reasons than that I love running and cycling. Adventure racing gets me out in the wilderness where I love to be. It makes me feel like an adventurer on an epic journey with a map."

Running fits into her life well as long as she does it first thing in the morning. Gina is typically very goal-driven, setting targets for four key areas of her life every year. In the past couple of years, a demanding job has left her struggling at times to find the right work-life balance. She decided to adjust her exercise goals. "When I was doing Ironman and running more seriously I was a lot more focused on my times, lap times, speed and speed training. Exercise was the No. 1 priority of my life during that time. It was very dominant and I loved it as that was the life experience I was seeking then. But I am not seeking that at this point in time. I am not as serious about my running as I used to be. At the moment it fits in really easily and keeps me off the wine and gets me to bed early. I like time to be structured so my exercise is quite a structured part of my life. My running is consistent when I have a goal. Without a goal, my running is not so consistent. I am always so mindful of my ITBs and injuries. I know if I run consistently I have to be equally committed to my rehabilitation activities and sometimes I just don't have the headspace to prioritise it all. I also go through periods where I am not interested in the pain I endure through the rehabilitation stuff I do such as massages."

Since Gina started running almost 20 years ago, she has found more reasons to run. "I would still say I run to feel free, get the high and to allow my mind to wander but I also run today to clear my head when I am stressed, because I love feeling fit and because I love spending time with my running girlfriends."

Gina cherishes the emotions of a great run which will boost her mood for the rest of the day. "I feel like I am solo, on an amazing yacht, sailing across the ocean on an incredible day with the wind in my hair."

Not every run feels that easy. "On bad days I feel heavy, slow, sluggish, like I have concrete legs. If I am training seriously for a race a bad physical run will mentally frustrate me. If I am not training seriously, then a bad physical run doesn't mean a bad mental one. If I consistently have bad runs it will de-motivate me and make me think there are other factors involved. If I have one bad run, it doesn't really affect my motivation – can't be perfect all the time."

Skipping sessions is part of the process and her response will depend on her goals. "It depends how mentally committed I am to running at that point in time. If I am heavily committed, I will get very frustrated with missing sessions for being sick or away. If running is not at the top of my priorities then I will miss it but I won't be hard on myself for doing so. I usually skip sessions when I am tired or have PMT."

She is more likely to run in a good mood. "But I will go for a run to shake a bad mood as I know what a positive release of negative feelings will occur if I go for a run. Running improves my physical wellbeing, my mental health, keeps me feeling positive and happy and grateful for the simple things in life."

Over the years she has found that running with others has great benefits. "I used to run alone for years but now I love running with my girlfriends and mixed groups. Now it means quality time with my girlfriends sharing something we all love. That is important to me. I talk about everything. It totally depends on who I am running with."

Gina has recommended others to take up running. "Lots of people think running is really hard. If you're starting from scratch you need to give yourself six months to experience the benefits of running. I recommend running groups to people, or I express the easy nature of running in that you just need a pair of sandshoes and off you go."

Gina's determination to find a solution for her injuries, refusing to believe that her running days were over in her early 20s, has allowed her to enjoy running and other sports again. Her decision to become a triathlete resulted in another life-changing event, meeting her fiancé Tony who has been a triathlete since his teens. Their home's third bedroom is set up as an indoor cycling studio which gets a lot of use. "Exercise in general has changed my life," Gina says.

CHAPTER 14
Running on a cruise boat was easier than we thought
"It is all about getting into a routine that you can maintain for the rest of your life."

Helen Bruce, 48, is a devoted runner and so is her triathlete husband Garry. The couple are creative at getting their training done, including during holidays that at first glance might not appear conducive to covering miles on foot, like boat cruises. "It was easier than we thought because on a cruise you can easily get into a routine, unlike other holidays when you are on the move every day on trains, planes and automobiles," Helen says.

"Every cruise has a different dynamic and this has an effect on the fitness environment. For example, our Mexican Riviera cruise was during the American school holidays and spring break, so there were lots of families and young adults on board. All were having a good time but there were also quite a few runners out each day. Our transatlantic cruise had an older demographic, with lots of well-travelled passengers in their 60s and 70s. It made us feel quite young at around 50. On this cruise, there were not so many runners but lots of walkers doing their daily routine."

Helen and Garry befriended the fitness instructors aboard their transatlantic cruise ship. "They said that on most cruises the fitness classes are full for the first two or three days with people keen to turn over a new leaf and get fit while on holidays."

With food flowing all day including midnight chocolate buffets and entertainment until the last person drops, few passengers stick to their cruise fitness plans, the instructors told Helen. The committed few on board, including Helen and Garry, could choose from an array of classes including aerobics, stretching, Pilates, yoga and personal trainer sessions. "Our favourite was the 7am stretching class, after our run. They also had the latest machines for running, cycling, rowing and lots of weights - both machines and free weights. Most people we met in the gyms were just maintaining their fitness while on the cruise rather than getting fitter, especially the runners," Helen says.

The trickiest part about running on a cruise ship is logging enough miles on the short jogging tracks. Most tracks have signs marking distance and the number of laps required for a kilometre and a mile. "It usually takes around four laps per kilometre or six laps to a mile. I found that I lost count of how many laps I had run so I tended to just run for time. It got a little boring at times but then you would find another runner to pace yourself with or look out to sea and daydream about all kinds of stuff."

Another challenge is finding a rhythm amid manoeuvring around the people who are walking on the track, as they typically outnumber those running. "Everyone has to go in the same direction of course or there would be chaos. Interestingly, people from different countries keep to a different side of the track. The Americans and Europeans tend to keep right as they would on the road in their countries, while others like us Aussies keep left. So you were never quite sure which way people would move. It was best if they just didn't move at all and we made our way around them," says Helen, adding that husband Garry managed to do speed sessions on the ship. "He would run at 90 percent when he had no one around and then use the heavy traffic times to recover for his next sprint."

Wind is a constant factor for a cruise runner. Windward running makes for excellent efforts, followed by a recovery when leeward. "The jogging track is usually on the top sports deck and is open to the weather. That is good when the weather is warm and nice in Mexico but not so good in the middle of the Atlantic Ocean when it's 8 degrees Celsius [46 degrees Fahrenheit] with a 30-knot wind and a rough sea."

While other decks on the ships might be better suited to running, restrictions apply to avoid runners pounding the decks directly above people's cabins.

The ship's movement is another variable to take into account. "When the weather was a bit rough you needed to be careful of your footing because quite often your feet did not land where you expected them to. A couple of times when the weather was really poor they closed the jogging track so we ran on the running machines in the gym, which was even trickier when the ship rolled. In fact a couple of times I thought I was going to slip right off the back of the machine. Thankfully I didn't."

Running proved an excellent topic to spark a conversation. "I believe that great holidays are made up of the people you meet and cruising is a wonderful way to meet new people. There was never much conversation on the jogging track. But later at the buffet or around the pool you would exchange running stories and fitness thoughts with someone you had seen on the track or in the gym, and learn about more great places to run and visit in the world. Or someone who did the daily Walk a Mile with the fitness instructors would see you going for the dessert tray and make a comment about you having to run twice as far the next day," Helen says.

Wearing her finisher's T-shirt from the 2007 Gold Coast marathon was the best invitation to a chat. "I met more people that day than any other day on holidays. People asked me if I really finished a marathon and what it was like. They wanted to know if the Gold Coast beaches are as nice as the travel shows say they are. As we are finding more and more, running makes our quality of life - even on holidays - that much better."

As a kid Helen enjoyed Little Athletics. As an adult she started running following the birth of her first son in 1982. "I found it an efficient way to lose some weight and gain some fitness without being away from home for long. I could do it anywhere anytime I had a babysitter - no flash running prams back in the early 80s. I guess I was inspired by my husband who had started running for fitness and also doing triathlons so it made sense to get some running shoes."

Running is now fully integrated into her life as well as that of Garry and their four sons. "Running has evolved into a whole lot more than just an efficient way to keep the weight under control and gain some fitness. It keeps me sane, it gives me time to myself - which is great when you have four sons in four years, it is an interest I share with my husband and it is a great way to see a new place when we are travelling. It also has a great way of solving any problems that may have arisen over the day. It is a great way to clear the head or come up with new ideas."

The lifestyle and fitness that come with being a runner are crucial for her. "Running is a big part of my life because it gives me a great sense of wellbeing in just about every aspect of my life. When I am feeling a bit down, a run will pick me up even though I might have to trick myself into getting out the door. When I am feeling great about life, I am usually fairly fit and running regularly. As I approach the age of 50 it gives me a level of fitness that allows me to remain active in all aspects of my life. I have read about the addictive qualities of endorphins and I guess I believe that. If for some reason I cannot run for a few days I definitely get irritable and struggle a little. Food can have the same affect, if I binge on junk food for a few days rather than eating a more healthy diet."

Over the years, their active lifestyle has also become an important part of their identities. Her husband and sons are very supportive of Helen's running, and vice versa. Friends and family also welcome their passion for running and triathlon. "My husband especially is supportive of my running and I am of his. It is definitely an important part of who we are as a couple and as individuals. Interestingly it is not something that we even thought about when we first got together 30 years ago. Our family is also very supportive of our running. Our friends are great about it as well and it often creates interesting conversation, especially when the guys start comparing fitness of footballers and triathletes."

Helen believes friends and family generally understand what running means to her. "But I think that even if they didn't, the fact that they support me and take an interest is enough."

Helen says her approach to running has changed since she took it up in 1982. "Most of the time I don't take my running as seriously as I used to when I was younger and now I just appreciate that I can run and wish to continue to do so. In contrast though, the training for my first marathon in 2007 definitely changed who I am and how I approach my running and fitness. I now know that I am capable of achieving anything I want to put my mind to and that my body is capable of adapting and handling so much more than I ever thought, especially if I look after it with rest and food. I gave up drinking alcohol for six months during my marathon training. Now that the drought is over I appreciate so much more how well I felt and my body functioned without drinking and with a structured training program.

"Running my first marathon under the guidance of Pat [Carroll] was truly a highlight of my life. The whole experience made me appreciate all those years of pounding the pavement, especially living in a remote part of Australia as we do."

She still learns about running every day. "I usually run five days a week and do not like to do less than this. I used to try to run every day but Pat pointed out to me that the benefit from my training was only as good as my recovery. So he taught me to have two rest days a week. I'm happy with that. It also makes sense as I get older. When I was running most days I was only maintaining 5km to 7km a day. Now with my rest days I manage to do more 10km, 14km and 21km runs over a month."

Helen has also become convinced of the benefits of keeping a written record of her training. "First of all, it validates the session and is great to look back on, especially if you record other things like effort applied, weather conditions, time of day, and even weight and blood pressure during serious training. These don't need to be too accurate but help to give you a good picture of what you have been doing. I especially found this helpful during my marathon training so that I could look back on the times I did for certain distances or certain interval sessions. It can be quite positive motivation as the history builds up. My husband has recorded every training session he has done for about 20 years. It is as good as a diary of his life showing when he has been sick or injured, when and where we have been on holidays, when he has been for a jog with me or one of our sons or a mate, and also any events he has competed in."

Helen now runs with a Polar heart rate monitor and downloads the data via its website. "This has been a great source of information for me which the website collates without me doing the math. For example it tells me I ran more than 1600km last year and trained an average of five sessions per week. It also monitors my heart rate and helps me to maintain a sensible pace especially if I am doing a 21km slow run for example."

Helen likes to start her days with a run, partly because it is the best way to ensure her training gets done. She says she is a morning person - she gets up at 3:30am to do her training. "It is also a great way to start the day. I am always full of beans when I get to work at 5am. I am a shift worker and work two 12-hour day shifts, two 12-hour night shifts, and then I have four days off. On some shifts I struggle to fit my runs in but generally my work suits my training fairly well."

Over the years Helen has recommended others to start running, but only after she has been asked for advice. "I rarely start this conversation because I feel it may intimidate people, even though I am just a social jogger. I often have conversations with women who run themselves down because they are not fit, are carrying extra weight or want to lead a more active lifestyle. I usually tell them that the chances of them winning a gold medal for Australia have probably passed so they don't need to get fit in a hurry. They should just look at doing something they can maintain for the rest of their life."

She advises budding runners to begin easy. "The best way to start running is to start walking. Then walk for two minutes, run for one minute. Then slowly, over weeks, you go a little further and a little further. I make sure they are aware of how slow you can run and how important it is to run slowly. I also tell them that initially it is all about how often they go, not how far they go. It is all about getting into a routine that you can maintain for the rest of your life."

CHAPTER 15
Running is my choice – and my success
"I used to run at 4:30am so no one would see me as I chased my dream."

Helen, who only wants her first name published, took up running in 2006 after three earlier attempts. She says she began to see if she could run a distance. "I am not sure what that distance was but I wanted to come back and say 'I have just been for a run'. I have always wanted to run. The image of *The Loneliness of the Long-Distance Runner* has always appealed. To me that image is of someone running the roads of Vermont among the autumn-coloured leaves. I've never been to Vermont," Helen says.

The painful experience of her relationship ending prompted Helen to finally commit to fulfilling her dream of becoming a runner. She followed a 10-week program that helped her build up to running for 30 minutes without stopping. She then put her newfound fitness to the test by entering Melbourne's 10-kilometre Run to the G. Finishing that race is her most cherished experience involving running. "I treasure the emotions of it all. It was tremendously cathartic. I was absolutely elated and could feel the tears welling up as I ran up the incline to whatever the bridge is that was the finishing stretch. I recall seeing the finish mark and feeling a power as if I was Cathy Freeman doing the 400 metres. I remember watching people who had finished long before me. Most were calmly walking back along the Yarra and I was thinking, `I'm one of them - I'm a runner'."

Having succeeded in becoming a runner meant a lot to her – it reminded her that she was able to achieve whatever she set her mind to without the help of anyone else, least of all the man who now no longer was a part of her life. "I was in Melbourne by myself. I had offered my former partner to come on the trip as mates and he mucked me around, refusing to commit or communicate. I had stayed on Collins Street where he and I had always stayed - it was a way to confront my past, accept it and move on. I had trained for this, my first-ever event, and was living the moment in a way that shocked me for its raw emotions. I knew my ex would have loved to have seen me complete the run, would have shared in my tears and would have been proud - after all, I wasn't really a runner. Our relationship was over, his affairs and our break-up were very raw. This was my way of proving to me I was someone who could achieve in my own right," she says.

"In reality I was already a very high achiever who has achievements many others are proud or envious of. I did this myself, from the training - I didn't train with Pat [Carroll] until after this event - to the interstate trip. People asked why I didn't do a run closer to home. It was deliberate at the time and in hindsight it was a test, a challenge. After the run, I walked to Myer for some food, with a red sweaty face and a drunken smile for everyone, feeling a tad strange. I was totally euphoric in the moment and cried, sobbing as I rang my family. The raw emotions of that time stay with me still and give me strength when I'm feeling vulnerable. I did it, myself, supported by me."

These days she runs because she can and loves it, as well as for general fitness. She has surprised a few people with beginning a commitment to running as an adult. "People are astounded, as I was known as a swimmer, not a runner."

Helen is now running two to three times a week, down from four to six times a week, to make time for other types of exercise including weights, swimming and cycling. She recently took up road cycling which she enjoys particularly during the hot summer months because she is able to stay cooler cycling than running. She also enjoys the fact that biking is easy on her joints.

Helen keeps track of her runs as she finds it very motivating. To Helen running means achievement of a dream, fitness, health and more freedom with her food. "I can more easily eat the calories," she says.

Running fits easily into her life, she says, especially now that she runs in a group. "When I started, I used to run at 4:30am so no one would see me as I chased my dream and I could do the solo running easily. Now it's easier to sleep in but the meeting-the-group concept gets me out of bed."

The people close to Helen support her passion for running, including her direct inspiration. "My former partner is thrilled for me and had always been encouraging of my attempts in the past."

Still, she doesn't think anyone really understands what running means to her. The people close to her say she has changed since she started running, "a bit madly obsessive," Helen says.

A great run lifts Helen's spirits and can boost her mood for hours. "I feel invincible, excited, strong, fit and healthy - until I see my red face. I have always gone beetroot-red with sport so it's not chasing glamour."

A session in which she struggles leaves her feeling disheartened, though pleased as well that she did run. "Once the endorphins kick in it doesn't really matter. Hopefully there's always the next run."

A run she is not happy with motivates her to train more or differently. "Varying the training is important."

Her running times, the time of day and the weather determine if she feels it has been a great run or the opposite. "I much prefer to run early morning in the cool before the rest of the early morning people are out and about. It's the solitude."

If she skips sessions she misses it. "And I find it stressful that I'm missing training. It's OK if I only miss up to six days - any more and it becomes a mental game to get back out there."

She's more likely to run in a good mood. A run always improves her sense of wellbeing. "I feel better, much better, no matter the type of run or the distance or the time," Helen says.

Running enhances her quality of life. "I feel better, more in control, stronger and sexier. My running is something that can only happen if I move my legs, at whatever speed - in my case slowly. So I am in control of going for my run: of reaching the bollards in under 15 minutes, or not; of getting to the gate that's the furthest I have ever run, or not; or deciding not to run but to walk. It's my choice, it's my success. For even though I might read lots for running education and information and have online coaching, it's still up to me to do it. The simple facts related to energy - it takes energy to run, why refuel on rubbish - have seen me lose weight in a consistent and maintained way and tone up. Hence I feel better, I feel stronger and it's directly related to my choices. I choose if, when and how I run. I choose what and when I eat and drink - I haven't become monastic. I'm in control, I'm not dependent or co-dependent, I'm me. I find independence and strength very appealing and subsequently a sexy attribute. If I feel good, sexy and confident, I'm sure I radiate that."

Helen says running is important to her health, adding that the sport has helped her to control her blood pressure. She considers herself to be healthier because she runs. Running is also important to Helen's self-esteem and self-image. "And that I keep running. Given that I was a late starter, I don't want to be seen as an adult giving up or having made a dumb choice to start a health activity and then give it up because it was all too hard."

She runs alone as well as with others. To her, the social aspect of running is not important, except for the motivation to get out of bed for training. "I love running by myself. It's very calming. I never use an iPod. I love running in a group but find myself ignoring requests to reply to chatter."

She signs up for an online program with Pat when she prepares for specific events. "I love Pat Carroll." Otherwise, a fortnight's plan is mapped out with her running group. Helen sometimes skips sessions from her training program because of "life-related fatigue". She won't feel guilty about doing so.

Since becoming a runner Helen has learnt to take care of her body and to stay aware of the signals it is giving her. She knows her shins will protest if she increases her training too much. "I currently have a bit of Achilles tightness that I'm being a bit cautious about."

Helen enters running races though she prefers to call them events. "To me racing infers a chance of winning, whereas I will never race in running. In running I am only competitive against myself but I have a very competitive nature in other sports."

Helen believes women approach running in a different way than men do. "[Women are] happier to go slower and are not as competitive. They are more supportive and encouraging."

Becoming a runner has changed her life in the sense that she gained confidence from achieving a dream, as she says, against all likelihood. She believes running is a lifestyle which she hopes to keep forever. Helen has made new friends because of running and doesn't think she has lost any because of it. "But a friend has. A friend now runs with me. She prefers to run earlier and the variety that we do. And her other friend has had a difficult time with this."

Helen has recommended many others to start running, including by handing out copies of the 10-weeks-to-30-minutes program she followed as a beginner. She even helped one runner through the program. "It's inspiring, motivating and great to see the results and achievements. Being a runner sets me apart in a positive, healthy role model, motivating, leadership kind of way. If I can do it anyone can but not that many do."

CHAPTER 16
I just didn't consider myself to be the sporty type

"The intensity and sacrifices involved in training for a marathon are all worthwhile when you realise, in the last 3km, that you are about to complete the biggest challenge of your life so far."

Karen Scott took up running at the age of 34 and realised she wasn't the un-athletic person she had always considered herself to be. Six years later Karen finished her first marathon at the Gold Coast in a better-than-expected 3 hours and 26 minutes. "The feeling of running down that finishers' chute brings tears to my eyes and makes my heart beat faster even now, two years later. It was euphoric. Nothing in my life has ever been close to that awesome feeling of achievement," Karen says.

That was July 2006 and Karen was on top of the world. But in February 2007, six months after achieving that milestone, a chronic hamstring injury stopped Karen from running and doing any exercise altogether. Only a year later, in 2008, was Karen slowly recovering from her injury with the help of experimental blood injection treatments. She has accepted and learnt to deal with the physical pain of her injury. But she's had a much tougher time with losing the ability to run and coping with the uncertainty of if, when and how she can return to the sport that has become a huge part of her life. "It has been the toughest 12 months, emotionally, that I have ever endured. I tried immersing myself more in work, trying other non-physically active hobbies, but nothing even comes close to what running gives me. Running is my identity - I am a runner. Without it I feel less than human. My confidence and self-esteem have taken a battering since I have been injured. I have suffered periods of depression, stress and emotional highs and lows. I have sought the help of a sports psychologist during this time, and he has helped a great deal, but I know that I won't feel real again until I am running again."

Despite initially being told her injury meant her running days were over, Karen is determined to return to the unlikely passion she only discovered in her 30s. "I used to be the queen of sleep-ins, although I was always conscious of my appearance. In high school I took up jogging on a bush track next to my family home but I'm sure this only lasted a number of weeks. I avoided sports carnivals at school and hated team sports, as I felt I didn't fit in and lacked the required skills to participate. I was the kid to always get picked last for a team; it was total humiliation which did nothing to boost my poor self-esteem at the time. I occasionally went through fads of taking up aerobics here and there, but that was about it. I weighed about 60 kilograms [Karen is 161 centimetres] within three years of getting married and thought I was just destined to be like that forever, because I didn't consider myself to be the sporty type."

Karen changed her mind – and body - when she and husband Neil bought a five-acre block of bush land in Martinsville, NSW, on the side of a steep ridge and started building their own home in 1997. At the same time she also began a low-fat diet. "To build our dream home - a pole home - we first had to clear the building site which meant some really hard yakka over many, many months. My body started to transform quite dramatically," Karen says.

In the three years it took the couple to build the house, Karen lost 7kg and gained plenty of energy. "I had never before been that slim and fit – I looked trim, taut and terrific and felt great. Every day was spent working on our hillside carrying heavy loads up and down, climbing, lifting, pushing a heavy wheel barrow and of course building the house."

When they finished construction in 2001, Karen took up walking and aerobics to preserve her newfound fitness. She also bought a slew of exercise equipment: a treadmill, exercise bike, elliptical trainer, rowing machine, aerobic step, gym ball, mini trampoline, weights, boxing bags, skipping rope and at least 20 exercise tapes.

In September 2001 she did a 40-kilometre charity walk, split into two 20km stretches over two days, along the shores of Lake Macquarie. "I felt alive, fit, healthy and keen to continue with my new way of life."

Karen decided to enter her first fun run the next month, the 5km Race for Research on the Newcastle foreshore. "My training consisted of seeing how far I could run, without stopping, the afternoon before the race. I did about 3km, with a very red face and a lot of puffing. So the following day I bravely fronted for the event all on my own and proudly completed it in 30:01. I felt so independent and proud of myself and with that I was hooked on running."

In 2001 Karen placed 51st out of 387 participants in the open female category. She has run that race every year since (except 2007 because of her injury). In 2006 she did a PB of 21:30 and placed 10th out of 620 women. "After doubting my athletic ability my whole life, I finally discovered that not only could I run, but for someone taking it up so late in life, I was quite good at it and competitive in my age group. It has developed into a passion that dominates my life. Nothing else can come close to matching the feeling I get when I run and compete."

Karen trained hard and enjoyed seeing her run times get faster. Besides running five times a week, she rode her mountain bike, did aerobics, weight training and used her other home gym equipment. She got her first age-group placing in 2003, finishing third in the hilly 5km Lindfield Fun Run in 23:51. She also ran her first half marathon that year. "I was so competitive, I couldn't wait to enter as many races as I could find that were within travel distance from home."

In 2004, she earned her first age-group win in the Wallaroo Fun Run near Raymond Terrace. "I was thrilled to finally achieve a gold medal that wasn't just for participation."

Besides numerous running races, Karen also entered cycling events with husband Neil. In 2005, Karen set her half marathon PB of 96:30 in Lake Macquarie.

And then came 2006. "Of course 2006 is the highlight of my running career so far being the Year of the Marathon. Sadly that is also what led to my long-term injury." Three earlier attempts to get to the start line of a marathon had failed, so finally being able to start and finish one meant a lot. Not to mention her fantastic time. "Nothing on earth could possibly feel better than achieving what only a year or two earlier seemed impossible. The intensity and sacrifices involved in training for a marathon are all worthwhile when you realise, in the last 3km, that you are about to complete the biggest challenge of your life so far. The high began when in the last 10km I ran past the pace group that I had thought I'd never be able to keep up with, and then finished four minutes ahead of them."

Karen was back training within two days after the Gold Coast marathon, doing brisk walks. She decided to run the Melbourne marathon, held three months later. "I began running again on the fifth day after the Gold Coast but was still too sore in the quads during the 6km jog. So I went back to walking for another couple of days before beginning a full week of running and cross-training again. Within seven days I was doing speed- and hill work, runs of between 8km and 14km, rode the exercise bike, lifted weights and did a 34km mountain-bike ride."

Eight weeks after her first marathon she was running more than 70km per week. Her longest runs were 36km which she did both in the ninth and tenth weeks. Then her body softly, but surely, started giving signs of protest. Karen sought treatment from her physiotherapist Brendan Clark, and acupuncture as well as weekly massage. "It was thought my problem was piriformis syndrome [a condition where the piriformis muscle irritates the sciatic nerve, causing pain in the buttocks and referring pain along the sciatic nerve] as my glute muscles were so tight and sore all the time."

She ran the Melbourne marathon in October 2006, finishing in 3 hours and 29 minutes. Again, she resumed training quickly. "I was regularly feeling pain in my left hamstring and both glutes but I still had only four days of complete rest. Within a week I was back to running, walking and cycling daily."

Early December, she finished the Tuggerah Lakes Festival half marathon in 1 hour and 40 minutes. The effort forced her to take a break from running. Instead, she did 10km walks and mountain-bike rides of up to two hours. "There was no way I was giving in and losing my fitness due to a pain in the butt. After 11 days of cross-training I tried a couple of 16km runs, but I was in pain a lot of the time. Despite this, on Boxing Day 2006 I began an advanced marathon training program while my injury steadily became worse.

"I was advised by Brendan to cut back on my running by initially eliminating my long runs, but I stubbornly kept running distances up to 21km. He then told me to cut out all speed work and hill work, as my injury wasn't responding to treatment and continued to get worse. I just wasn't listening. Despite taking his advice by this time, I was still doing far too much and not listening to the signs my body was giving me. I eventually had to concede defeat and give up running altogether on February 19, 2007, when I got only 1km into a morning training run and broke down in pain. Even then, instead of walking home I jogged - talk about stubborn. By now I had a sports physician, physiotherapist, acupuncturist and massage therapist all trying to work out why my piriformis was giving me so much trouble and why it wasn't responding to any form of treatment."

In May 2007, she went to Sydney where an MRI showed a small tear in her left hamstring, bone marrow oedema at the junction of both hamstrings and bilateral hamstring tendinitis. Her physio referred her to Brent Kirkbride, a sports physiotherapist at the Sydney Sports Medicine Centre. "Brent told me that he had treated several long distance runners around my age with this type of injury but mine was the worst case he had seen. He gave me little hope of ever running more than 10km again, but even that would take many, many months to achieve. I was devastated, heart broken, angry and lost. I couldn't believe that I, an ordinary runner without any special ability, could possibly end up with such a serious injury."

She was given a series of glute and hamstring strengthening exercises and nerve stretches. It was almost all she could do, as by then her hamstrings had become too painful to do any form of exercise. Initially she had continued her cross-training. "In February, when I was forced to stop running, I still believed it would just be a matter of weeks before I could run again. I started circuit training, skipping, high energy aerobics, and aqua aerobics and rode many kilometres on my mountain bike to try to compensate for the loss of running time and to desperately avoid gaining weight. I still ignored any signs that my legs were getting sorer, believing that any day they would start to show improvement: after all, I was no longer running and that is what caused the problem in the first place."

She decided to take took swimming lessons too. At first she could barely do one 25-metre lap, but within six weeks she could do 26 laps. "I was so proud of myself that I deemed 2007 to be the Year of the Swim. I felt that my injury must have been fate, just so I could finally learn to swim. However, all this was done without kicking, instead using a pull buoy and flippers for flotation."

But it aggravated her injury and Karen had to stop swimming seven weeks after she started. "My hamstrings, particularly the left one which had the tear, were just so sore that I couldn't bend over, sit for more than 10 minutes or walk up stairs without pain. I couldn't even go outside for a short walk."

In August 2007, Brent told Karen about experimental autologous blood injections which had mostly been used in Melbourne to treat AFL players with similar injuries. Your blood has growth factors that can help healing in injuries of muscles, tendons and ligaments. These growth factors may lessen pain and disability and speed the recovery from injury. Karen had the procedure done on her left leg. "Blood was taken from my arm and, guided by ultrasound, was immediately injected into the left hamstring after a local anaesthetic. After three weeks of total rest and five more of light exercise, my left leg was starting to feel less sore and I was gradually able to begin riding and doing aerobics again."

By January 2008 she could do three-hour mountain bike rides, lower body weights and even a few jogs of about 3km. Then she suffered another setback. "My right hamstring had started to become worse. So in mid-February, one year after first breaking down, I had blood injections into both hamstrings."

About a month after the procedure, Karen was able to ride the exercise bike, do upper body weights, and her leg and glute exercises. "My right leg is still quite painful and aches whenever I drive or sit for long periods. It will still be months before I can again try some short jogs but my physiotherapists are hopeful that I will be able to run short distances again one day. It sadly seems my passion for long distance running may never again be realised. I have been told to aim for triathlon instead, as it isn't as hard on the body. At the moment I'd just be happy to be able to walk out the door and do a slow 5km jog," Karen says.

Dealing with her injury has been hard. "During the last 12 months I have felt very lost, sorry for myself, miserable and low. I still haven't found anything that comes even close to filling the space that not being able to run has left in my daily life. It was a major part of a very active lifestyle and I miss it terribly. I ache when I see other people out running on my way to work. When travelling my favourite running routes I often wonder if I'll ever get to run them again."

She sought help from sports psychologist Paul Penna. "He has really helped me in dealing with my injury and my future – possibly in triathlon. I can't thank him enough: I am in a completely different and much happier headspace now compared to six months ago. He has helped me come to terms with the changes in my body since giving up running, which are really hard to accept. The emotional issue of injury is like a grieving process that takes time to work through. All my goals were running related and based on marathons and even ultras in the future. I now know that won't be possible. I feel that if I had listened to advice in the early stages of the running injury, it wouldn't have become as chronic as it did. If only I had taken weeks instead of days to rest properly after my first marathon. Hindsight is a wonderful thing. I've certainly learnt my lesson the hard way. If only I'd listened to my body when it started to feel tired and sore I'd probably still be running."

While she will have to adjust her long-term running goals from marathons and beyond, to shorter runs and triathlons, she remains determined to run again. "Running has made me more confident, self-assured, independent, more driven and passionate. It has certainly changed my life dramatically, to say the least."

(This story first ran in Australia's *Run For Your Life* magazine)

CHAPTER 17
Effort and commitment lead to surprising results

"Running gives me confidence to be true to myself and reminds me to push my own limits regularly, both on the road and in life in general."

Karey Corrie, now 29, had been running intermittently since high school. Recently she decided to make a commitment to her run training. "Sport was always a big part of my life and has stayed with me into my adulthood. I only started running more seriously about 18 months ago. I had wanted to regain my fitness as I struggled to find some direction in my life and running had always been something I enjoyed so I decided to set a goal and get myself moving again. I was at a crossroads and needed something to focus on to help move me forward. Despite my inconsistency in previous years, running had always been there for me and proven quite therapeutic, so I set a goal and went from there. I felt that if I could become a runner again it might help boost my confidence and help me along my journey," Karey says.

Karey has since found additional motivation to run and to make her goals more challenging. "Running has become my daily therapy I suppose. I have come to rely on the regular training to help me stay grounded and in tune with myself, not to mention the stress release through exertion and the fabulous and addictive endorphin rush. My goals have changed. They are bigger now and it is in that way that running has taught me to continue to stretch my boundaries, to constantly challenge myself and that with consistent effort and a genuine commitment you can achieve things you may once have never thought possible."

Running is Karey's favourite way to exercise. "I prefer running because of the simplicity, the solitude sometimes and the connection it allows me to have with my running friends and even running strangers. I also love the idea that my progress or performance is completely up to me – what I get out is what I put in."

Karey runs four times a week following an online training program designed for her specifically by Pat Carroll. She keeps track of her sessions. "I would love to run every day but I know rest is just as important as the quality speed or distance session. Before I started with Pat online I would use a training diary but I was never consistent for more than a few months. Now, though, I record every session and send it through to Pat at the end of each week."

She enjoys having a training schedule tailored to her ability and goals, and sticks to it. "It helps to keep me moving in the direction I want to be going and focused on achieving my goals. I only skip if I am injured or there has been a death in the family."

She rewards herself for consistent training and reaching certain goals. "I look at each training session as money in the bank – each session is worth $5. At the end of the month I treat myself to a new running shirt or other running gear. Sometimes I save up over a few months for big items but whatever I get is all about adding to my motivation for running."

When she has to skip a few sessions, she misses her training and feels guilty. "I get cranky and frustrated and impatient. I find the motivation easy to get back. I am usually rearing to go. But physically I usually find it will take a week to be feeling as good as I did before being sick or injured, depending on how long I was off for. I was recently injured and had missed two sessions over four days. I hated myself for it even though I had been advised not to run until all pain was gone. It does not make sense but that is how I felt."

To Karey, running means freedom, accomplishment, hard work and routine. "It also means my health and a better ability to chase after the kids. My running is a habit now and a regular part of my daily and weekly schedule. I work my runs in around my work and family commitments and combine them where possible."

The people close to Karey are supportive of her passion for running. "My partner in particular always cheers me on and will attend events with me, encourages me on low days and always makes wonderful comments like, `You have such great runners' legs', when I have one of those days where I wonder why I am doing it all and whether it is all worth it. My mum is also really supportive. She often joins me on my easier runs and has now started training for some events herself."

She believes her loved ones understand what running means to her. "My partner and my mum certainly do. They know I am a much more contented person with running in my life."

They say Karey has changed since she began running. "My partner thinks I am more relaxed and have more of my normal sense of calm compared to when I am not running. Personally I also feel more focused when I am running compared to not running."

When Karey has a great run, she feels like she can do anything. "That life is great and the world is my playground to explore one kilometre at a time; confident in myself and my abilities; and that, if nothing else, I have accomplished one great thing for the day."

When her run is a struggle occasionally, Karey says she feels depressed. "Then I have lots of self-doubt: why am I doing this; I'm really not very good at it; I should just give it away; and I feel cranky and do not want to talk."

Both mental and physical aspects determine whether she feels it has been a great run or a bad one. "Probably the mental side has more bearing because it would be my perception of the physical exertion or effort that contributed to the feeling of a good run versus a bad run. Also sometimes I am pretty hard on myself mentally. Sometimes distance and time play a part too, in that if I have made my time goal or my goal distance then it was good and if not then it was bad. But this really comes back to the standards I set and my mental approach to achieving them in that session."

A great run will boost Karey's mood for at least a day. If she is not happy with her training she can usually find something positive about it after a few hours. "I have not forgotten by the next session but I have used it to learn what I can do better for the next session."

She always feels better after a run and she doesn't let her mood affect her decision to train. "I am equally motivated to run when feeling good and actually rely on my running when in a bad mood because I know it will help me to snap out of it."

Running has lifted her quality of life. "Life is much sweeter when I am running. I appreciate the small things more when I have running to allow me time to reflect on them."

Karey considers running vital to her health. "It keeps me active and mobile, maintains my cardio function and sets a great example for my kids to be healthy. I consider running an important part of staying healthy but it is not the only factor."

It is also very important for her self-esteem. "Self-image I am OK with but confidence is an ongoing battle for me – running is like a little rocket booster in this area."

She does two of her weekly training sessions alone and the other two with a friend. "I love to run alone for the escape and the solitude but I also love running with my running buddy. Sometimes we don't talk at all but just knowing she is there beside me keeps me going. I run for myself mostly. I do enjoy the buddy sessions and fun runs so I guess the social aspect does play a part."

When Karey runs with her friend they discuss a range of topics. "Usually our chats are relatively serious – personal problems, world issues. Other times they can be quite light. Mostly though we help each other sort through issues on the run, if we have enough energy and breath to talk that is. I feel that the camaraderie and connection that develops between women through running is a bigger part of their running than it is for men. That aspect of connectedness through continuous forward motion over time is something special as we learn more about each other, our families and our hopes and dreams, not to mention solving the problems of the world on the run."

She has recommended others to take up running. "I get them to run with me in a fun event and then ask them to join me on some training runs and keep encouraging them."

Races inspire Karey's training. She is currently training for a marathon. Her favourite running experience so far is finishing her first half marathon. "The whole race was incredible, from the view to the spectator support and the way I actually felt on the day. It was a perfect run."

She says she is competitive. "Mostly I am competing against myself in running and also in other areas of life. I set high standards for myself and I am constantly trying to achieve them whether running or at work. My competitiveness is relative to the goal I have set for myself rather than who else is running and how fast they are going."

Becoming a runner changed Karey's life. "I feel more confident. I am more organised. I manage stress better. For such a simple activity, running gives me a myriad of benefits. The most important thing for me is that running gives me confidence to be true to myself and reminds me to push my own limits regularly, both on the road and in life in general."

She plans on remaining a runner as long as she likes being one. "I have not set an age limit. I will continue for as long as I can find new challenges and continue to enjoy it."

CHAPTER 18
I'll keep running until I find an age group I can win
"Races gave me the motivation to keep running. I kept every certificate, timing list and T-shirt from the first few years."

Katrina Crook began running as a teenager because she wanted to shed a few pounds. She didn't particularly enjoy it and found little motivation at a time when the sport didn't have the popularity it does now. After she became a mum at the age of 25, she resumed running because she needed the fitness for playing soccer. She still didn't like it. It was not until she did a race a few years later that she found all the motivation she needed - and then some.

Katrina is now 39 and loves being a runner. "Originally I ran as a way of dieting as a young girl but I hated it. Back then it wasn't a popular sport and I don't remember any real information, especially running stores, being out there. Without races for motivation it was an on/off thing for many years. After the birth of my first child I took up playing soccer as a way of losing the baby fat. I enjoyed that but I needed to keep fit so I took up running again. Even then I only really ran enough to be able to play soccer and still wasn't really enjoying it as such. Therefore, running was still an on/off affair for some years."

Katrina joined a gym when her children started school and attended the local gymnastics centre. "I figured I could exercise while they were at gymnastics. After several months of running on the treadmill I had the opportunity to enter what was then the Bridge to Bay and is now the Bridge to Brisbane. I loved it and never really looked back from then. Races gave me the motivation to keep running. I kept every certificate, timing list and T-shirt from the first few years."

Katrina just ran, without a coach or training program. "I got no advice nor did I seek any out about running. I got on a treadmill every day - yes 7 days a week - for months. I really honestly believed that I could lose fitness overnight if I didn't. It wasn't until a forced layoff one week out from my first race that I really saw the benefits of rest or tapering. I wish I had more knowledge when I started. I wish I knew what I know now."

Katrina has become a different runner since she began entering races. "My reasons for running have changed a lot. I wish I had discovered a passion for running a lot earlier. Back then you could do a race every weekend over the winter period. I entered almost every run going. I got into half marathons very early on and discovered a love for distance running. I loved the training time and saw it as me-time leaving two young kids at home. With a very supportive partner I had no trouble getting out of the house.

"Now I love the sense of fitness and accomplishment that comes with running. I love that I can run for three hours and still pull up fine that afternoon. I love that I'm not out of breath participating in activities with my kids, both as a school teacher and a mother. I love the fact that people think I'm mad for even contemplating a half hour run let alone a full marathon which I took up two years ago. I love that I can decide to join people I've never met on a weekend away running just because I'm fit enough to do it. I did this recently with a group I met online on Coolrunning."

Katrina participates in triathlon as well but prefers running. "I always say that triathlon would be a great sport without the swim and the bike. Perhaps it's the simplicity of running. All you need to run is a good pair of shoes, and perhaps a great sports bra, in order to get out there and do it. Triathlon is a lot of time spent making sure you have a ton of the right gear needed to make it through the three disciplines. Running is me, an iPod and my thoughts for hours on end. What more could you want?"

These days Katrina aims to run five times a week, varying distances. "I am consistent with it as long as the motivation is there. If I have a race coming up and a training plan, I am much better at getting out there. Without a race in sight I can be a bit naughty and put it off, finding too many excuses."

She keeps track of her training in a log book. She often uses training programs provided on race websites. "I can be quite anal about this. I love having a plan and boxes to tick off. I tend to use more online tracking systems these days. For the first few half marathons I downloaded the training plan from the website, printed it out and dutifully did every run filling in the boxes, keeping a record of heart rate etc. For the marathon this year, the plan comes as a PDF-file you can save and tick the little boxes on screen - very exciting."

When Katrina started doing triathlons, her husband soon followed suit. He then weighed about 125kg. "As an ex-state swimmer he soon got back into the swimming side of things and then took up the riding with a passion. To date he has around six bikes in the house all with a different purpose - or so he tells me. Since first taking up triathlon he has lost around 40kg and weighs in at just over 80kg."

In 2007 her husband did his first Ironman, which involves swimming 3.8km, cycling 180.1km before running a 42.195km marathon, and loved it. "The volumes of training are large. He is out almost every weekend for hours on end and out very early on the weekday mornings. Large parts of my weekend mornings are now long runs. Weekdays are only 40 to 60-minute runs."

The active couple's children are 13 and 15 respectively. "We find a way to fit it all in. I am often left to get the children ready for school in the mornings, though they are now a lot more independent in this regard, and on my own on the weekends. But it's what we want to do and we make it work. We support each other 100 percent in our goals and it's important that we are able to do these things."

Katrina says that support from loved ones is crucial. "I feel quite sorry for people doing it without the support of partners. When we are together we make it count. This is starting to sound like we never see each other but we do. We love what we do, we support each other and we make it all fit. It's not all bad. I got a holiday to New Zealand while he did an Ironman, we went trail running at Binna Burra together on our 20th wedding anniversary with a group of people we'd only ever met online, and we had many other holidays away with the family chasing races. If I had the money I would swan around the world in an attempt to complete every marathon there was."

Their non-running and non-triathlon friends question their sanity, though they have met many like-minded runners and triathletes through their active lifestyle and made new friends. She believes that the friends who are not involved in endurance sports don't understand what running means to her. "I don't ever think that a non-runner can really understand what running means to someone who does run, especially those of us who choose the distance stuff."

Since she and her husband became active participants in running and triathlon their social life has expanded. "We have met quite a number of people through racing and training. My husband is involved with an Ironman group and they encourage partner support through regular get-togethers. It's not unusual at a race now to be looking and waiting for about 20 people to cross the finish line. We have a core group that we have met through triathlon and running. We now go away together. We go to dinner together – it helps that everyone is ready to leave or go to bed by about 9pm. At races we now set up a marquee together and cheer on husbands or wives. It makes a lovely social day. We make new friends through the old friends. The list keeps growing. It's important for the whole family to be involved, not just those running or racing. Knowing people at the races is great otherwise it can be a very lonely day for those on the sidelines."

Katrina's parents encourage their lifestyle. "My parents are supportive and often have the children while we go away racing. They came to watch my husband in his first Ironman. My mother's greatest fear, though, is that I will die while racing. I can't convince her otherwise. It seems that she is happy for my husband to race the longer distances, just not me."

Katrina says she is healthier and happier since she and her husband made their lives more active. "It's a lifestyle change. This is where I am lucky that we have a shared passion. We are doing it together. We are motivated. We support each other. Life is great."

Being a distance runner is a lifestyle. "Timetabling is involved just to fit everything in. We are essentially morning people, used to getting up at 4am or 5am to train and then falling asleep on the couch or floor at 8pm. If the whole family wasn't involved you could begin to resent the intrusion it makes on your life."

She truly appreciates the runs that feel great, even more so after a forced layoff because of injury. "That feeling you get when you know you've achieved something else that run is hard to describe. You know you ran well and the data proves that when you download your watch. The feeling that you get when you cross the line in a time you didn't expect - absolute elation.

"I had a knee operation for torn cartilage last year and was out for months. It has given me a renewed appreciation of running. It's so hard to not be able to run. I ran on my knee just before the operation last year in a half marathon which I'd paid for before I knew about the operation. I hurt all the way but I crossed the line in under two hours beyond all my expectations. I'd pushed myself really hard, I'd run on Nurofen - yes I know very naughty - but I'd done it. My husband kept bobbing up around the course to cheer me home."

Those sessions or races that she is not happy with, she just forgets. "I don't worry too much about crap runs. Draw a line, move on, tomorrow's another day. After the knee operation if I feel like quitting I remember what it's like to not be able to run. I'll get out there again."

She believes the difference between feeling that it was a great or a bad session is mental. "I tell people that running is 90 percent a head game. If you can conquer your head you've already won. I went out for a run this week after I hadn't been doing a lot over the past fortnight. I started off slow, told myself to push it and did. I ran strong and came home strong. I felt good."

While she easily finds excuses to skip a run, she also finds it easy to get back into a routine. "After the knee operation I was out for four months. I nagged the physio every week to run again. She said no. I did really miss it because I couldn't. That was hard. I was in the middle of marathon training and I knew I was losing fitness. Once I got the go ahead I was back running long weekend runs within a month. I found it easy to get back into it because it's what I wanted to do and I had been forced out."

Katrina definitely feels better after a run than before. "I come home ready to face the day, awake and alert. I feel better through the day if I've run that morning. I sometimes use running as a way to improve a bad mood. I love the solitude and thinking time."

She considers her running very important to her health. "Because ill health means a day off running, I need to keep myself healthy. I rarely have a day off work because I try hard to maintain good health. I may jinx myself here but I am rarely unwell. I don't consciously think about the health benefits but I do try to maintain good health."

She is unsure about the impact being a runner has had on her self-esteem and self-image. "I do feel good about the fact that I can run. I often don't even see myself as a runner. I see runners as those with the long legs out there winning the races. I see myself as someone who enjoys running. I know that I feel fatter etcetera when I'm not running but this is probably more of a woman thing. My body image is different when I run to when I don't."

Katrina likes running alone and with others. "I love the solitude but running with a group pushes me to run faster and I need that. I get too used to plodding along. I love to run with my husband. Although he is faster than me it's nice to get out together. I hate running with new groups as I worry I will slow them down. If I run with a group I need to know them first. I don't have any girlfriends who would run with me. They'd all laugh at the idea. Any girlfriends within our running circle are supporters rather than participants. If I run with anyone it is usually my husband's training partners and friends. They are all male and all into Ironman and so all faster than me. I am definitely at the back. Besides, if I get a choice of which group to run with I will take the faster group and then push myself but it does mean that I am usually at the back."

Katrina only follows training programs if she is preparing for a half marathon or a marathon. "It gives me the confidence that I am doing it properly and can race well on the day. It gives me the motivation to train. For races between 5km and 10km I just get out there and run."

Katrina says she is competitive in the sense that she aims to improve her own times. "The only competition in running is against me. I never enter a race thinking that I am going to win. I know that I place in about the top third of the field and that's where I like to stay. The only time I'm trying to beat is my own. I have certain goals and PBs that keep me motivated to train and race. I can get competitive in the race itself in trying to pass the person in front, then the next one in front but I know I'm not going to win. I don't think I am competitive in my career. I have a great job as a teacher but I'm not aspiring to move through the ranks." Katrina's ultimate goal is to complete a 100km race. "That will come, the time just isn't right yet."

Katrina realises her sport comes at a price but she finds that the rewards far outweigh the cost. "I know I'm fitter than I was 15 years ago. Running gets me outdoors and doing something. It keeps me motivated. I know I've spent far too much money over the years on shoes, outfits, doctors and physio bills. Perhaps I'd be a lot richer without running in my life but I'm not sure I'd be happier. I am keen to be involved in any activity that requires a level of fitness. I love any new sports and will do just about anything. Running gives me the fitness to do that."

She hopes to keep running for many years to come, perhaps even for glory. "I joke and say that I'm going to keep running until I find an age group I can win. Seriously though, I will keep running until I physically or mentally can't do it any longer. I would love to still be running at 60 or 70 but I fear that injury may stop me before then."

So far Katrina is going strong. She credits the physiotherapist who has helped her physically and mentally through two main injuries that prevented her from running. "I have a terrific physio who I know I could not do this without. I have been with her forever. When I tore the ligaments of my ankle she was the one who assured me that I would run again. I tell her that she saved my life. It took doctors eight months to discover what she knew in a week. Without her I may have given up long ago. She understands my need to run and rarely tells me no. She simply finds a way to make it work for me."

CHAPTER 19
Take control of your destiny by going for a run
"For all its connotations with discipline and routine, it is a very user-friendly and flexible sport requiring minimum props and expense."

Keryn Clark started running in June 1982 when she was in her mid 20s. Back then she was a 40-a-day smoker and in very bad shape. Watching her brother compete in the 89-kilometre Comrades Marathon in South Africa, where Keryn lived at the time, she decided it was time for a change. "Standing there with a cigarette in my hand and feeling dreadful I looked at all these people finishing and thought that this was something I wanted to do. I put the cigarette out there and then, and took up running the moment I arrived back in Johannesburg. People laughed at me because I was famous for my lack of discipline and bad habits but I stuck with it. The memory of those Comrades runners finishing was a defining moment for me. Within 10 days I walked, limped and jogged my first road race," Keryn says.

More than a quarter century later Keryn is still a runner and lives accordingly. "I don't have the same lifestyle - my old one would have killed me decades ago. However I am an addictive person and I get bored easily. Running helps me maintain a balance and sets up the day for useful activity."

She prefers running over other exercise. "I just can't get enthusiastic about other sports. I've tried them all. I loathe the gym. Running, for me, is the best sport because you can take it anywhere and it doesn't need a lot of paraphernalia to get going. You just need the will and a pair of shoes and you can run all over the world with it."

She now runs four to five times a week consistently. She always keeps track of her sessions, a habit she got into when she started in June 1982. She has 26 log books, one for each year of running.

Running is essential to Keryn. "It means everything. It is important for maintaining a balance and keeping me positive about life. It's fun and it feels good. Running has always been a priority. While I am not as obsessive as I used to be, everything I do has to accommodate my running."

For Keryn running boosted the quality of life. "I shudder to think where I would be if I hadn't found running. Running not only gives health benefits, but the whole superstructure of running comes with friends, trips away and planning for events. Running is a lifestyle, not something tacked onto the beginning or the end of one day in a life. When I look back the memories that stand out in technicolour are the running ones and the friends I made along the way."

Running is very important to her self-esteem and self-image, Keryn says. "Apart from the obvious overt health benefits, like a slim physique, there are the emotional and mental benefits about taking control of your life, making decisions to be active when you don't want to be. Racing is a great teacher in studying form, in thinking on your feet, in extracting from yourself a pound of flesh and metering it out, one kilometre at a time for best effect. All these skills and abilities are activated quietly when you run or race and as they develop so does your self-esteem. I get bored easily and one of the negative results of that boredom when I was young was bad lifestyle choices. Good or bad choices work in tandem with self-image. When positive choices are made, self-image is lifted."

Running always improves her frame of mind. "By going for a run you take charge of your destiny and control is back in your hands. That becomes an empowering tool which lifts any mood."

The people close to Keryn are supportive of her passion for running and she believes they definitely understand what running means to her. Her loved ones say she has changed since she took up the sport. "My brother got me into running. He has seen me become a lot more focused, more positive and more structured in my approach to life. I also make healthier lifestyle choices."

Her decision to start running has been crucial to her health. "At 24 I was washed up from too many cigarettes, too much alcohol, partying, drugs and bad food. I could not walk up a flight of stairs and emotionally I was very fragile. I could very easily have been one of those young people who are found dead from an overdose."

In many ways Keryn considers herself to be healthy because she runs. "Although, having said that, you can't assume that running is the balm for all ills. Along with the commitment to running comes the commitment to give your body the best chance of running at its best and this requires attention to the details of sleeping well, food, drinking water and no cigarettes."

The change in lifestyle also meant a different social life: Keryn has made new friends because of running and lost touch with old ones. "Running involved a 360-degree lifestyle change for me. I no longer stood in smoky clubs at 3am on a Saturday night. I became boring to my old friends and they became boring to me. Looking back I wouldn't have changed it for the world."

Keryn typically trains by herself. "Generally I prefer running alone or with an in-sync partner who also likes to run lost in their own thoughts. I turn up my iPod and meditate while I am running. The social aspect of running is very important after the event, but in training and racing I go it alone."

Keryn says she loves training programs, with one caveat. "I just never follow them. I listen to my body. If it's tired and I have a long run scheduled, I won't do the run or I will shorten the session. Sometimes my body just doesn't want to do what the schedule says. The trick is to understand the difference between a tired body and the mind being lazy. When I have followed training programs to the letter I've done very well."

Keryn won't let her mood affect her decision to run, though to do so in a bad one requires more willpower. "When I am depressed I have to force myself out of the door."

A great session or race leaves Keryn feeling light, positive and in control. "All the cogs are oiled and the wheels are turning smoothly. A good run in the morning will boost my mood for a day, a PB for a whole week and a marathon PB could boost my mood for a month."

A session during which she struggled used to feel like the end of the word. "These days a crap run is a disappointment, particularly if it happens during a race, but I'm more pragmatic.

There are swings and roundabouts in running. I know that a crap run will be followed by a great one and visa versa. You just take it on the chin and keep going. Generally I will be inspired to train harder. I wouldn't skip sessions in protest."

Both mental and physical factors determine whether she feels it has been a great run or a bad one. "If my body feels like I am moving cement under water then it's a crap run. However sometimes you can feel crap for the entire run and still manage a PB. I guess a crap run is when you have not met your own expectation for the run. It's then that you need to remind yourself that simply being able to be out running is a gift in itself."

In her running Keryn competes against herself and the clock. She does draw inspiration from fellow runners, like she did in a 10km race in London, UK. "It was a three-lap course and she and I were evenly paced. The lead between us changed several times. To beat her I had to dig deeper than I had ever gone. Coming down the final straight she was a hair's breadth in front and I thought that it was now or never. I surged and held my breath all the way to the finish and triumphed. I had run PBs at 5, 8 and 10km. After the finish we looked at each other too tired to speak but we each knew that we had tested the other to the core. We shook hands without a word and walked off into our respective lives. I have never forgotten her or matched those PBs."

Keryn believes women take a different approach to running than men do. "I think women have more to juggle than men and for this reason their time has to be properly managed. I have heard coaches say that when women become serious they are more focused than men and they make tougher competitors because a woman's life is all about endurance, tolerance, patience and mental toughness.

"Women also don't have those bursts of testosterone which makes them rush to the front in a big show of one upmanship. But don't let an apparent lack of action fool you - women have patience. I can't tell you the number of men who have screeched past me with a great show of bravado in races, who I have relentlessly stalked, just waiting for the right moment to pick them off and sail past without batting an eyelash."

She has recommended others to start running. "I make suggestions to new people and give them a magazine or a pair of shorts. If they want to do it, they will. My favourite running protege was an African colleague who was rather large. At that time in South Africa, African women did not participate in running. We were trying to get a relay team together for the office and I gave my friend a pair of my running shorts to encourage her to start. She did not participate in the relay but years later wrote to me to say running had changed her life. In her own time and her own place she had donned the shorts and trained in her own way. She has since run 12 Comrades Marathons."

The single-most important thing about running for Keryn is its flexibility. "For all its connotations with discipline and routine, running is a very user-friendly and flexible sport requiring minimum props and expense. With the exception of shoes you come equipped with all you need; legs, a heart and a mind. The experience and the poetry of running is how the three integrate at any given time."

CHAPTER 20
A desire to run drove my successful rehabilitation

"It's a source of satisfaction and personal achievement that's always with me, no matter how other aspects of my life might be faring."

Lisa Hurring began running at the age of 29 in April 2006 because it was something she had always wished to do. She was a competitive swimmer looking for a new challenge - Lisa has been swimming since the age of seven. "I had always admired those who seem to effortlessly cover ground as they run. It seemed a kind of meditation to me, to be out there with a fit body in the fresh air and sunshine and no mechanical aid at all to assist you. I also desperately needed a new challenge. Having been a swimmer for over two decades and no squad to train with here, I was bored swimming alone and feeling anyway that there was nothing new to learn in that sport. I really needed to move into something new. The time was finally right for me to start running and I became addicted very quickly," Lisa says.

But seven months later Lisa's leg was shattered in a motorbike accident. Facing a long and painful rehabilitation, a return to running became Lisa's primary goal. "Before I broke my leg I had a knee issue that stopped me running for a month – I thought my world was ending. I was dying to get back in my shoes and it definitely made me more determined to run. When I broke my leg a short time later, running was all I could think about and my whole rehab was done with the eventual goal of running again in mind. That's a big part of why I worked through it so hard – I just wanted to run again."

That desire made her determined to succeed – which she did faster than anyone had predicted. "It was a massive part of my recovery in terms of aims and pushing me to work hard. If I'd not had the running to work for and just the vague need to recover sometime, I'd never have done as much as I did."

During her recovery Lisa couldn't bear to read her running magazines for three months. "I got straight into rehab while still in hospital and kept the thought of returning to running at the very forefront of my mind all the time but it was just too much to be reading of races and training tips when I couldn't even walk."

Before her accident Lisa felt very competitive about her running. "When I first started and then began training with an online coach to reach 10km performance goals I hadn't really changed at all at that point. I did feel calmer and very satisfied within myself after a good run but my competitiveness and drive to do better had increased a lot. I remember this strange mix of feelings on a good run of partly wanting to relax and enjoy the feeling, and partly wanting to concentrate on beating my time and thinking of goals."

Her ability to overcome the obstacles she faced following her accident has strengthened her self-confidence and self-belief. "My determination to get back to running in terms of pushing myself through rehab constantly is a major part of that. Dealing with constant and often very severe pain for most of the first few months of my rehab has made me stronger. I remember laughing out loud during one particularly sore day of walking with my crutches because I'd remembered whinging during countless swimming sessions at feeling tired or achy or lazy and wanting to just get out and go home to be a normal kid. I also remembered how frustrated I had been two months before breaking my leg when a knee niggle put me out of running for two weeks - there's nothing like a little perspective to put those niggles in their place."

Lisa says her personality changed because of the challenges she had to conquer during her rehabilitation. "Before the accident I was highly strung, my competitive drive was far too high and as a result I was getting overly frustrated and disappointed in small setbacks. Those little setbacks and perceived failures often knocked me flat because I was very much lacking in self-confidence. This was reflected in other areas of my life too, with a big example being my reluctance to stand up and address work concerns due to weakness and a habit of avoiding any conflict as much as possible. Now I am far stronger and I remember feeling really surprised when first noticing these changes during a work discussion. I was no longer afraid and the work issue was just that – a work issue. Once we'd talked about it, it was over and I felt fine. I wasn't worked up and upset over it as I once would have been because from my new perspective I could see the issue for what it was, just another little niggle. I'd shown myself through that hard rehab that I was more than capable of dealing with obstacles far larger and more fearsome than some niggle."

She cherishes her accomplishments as an athlete, and particularly as a runner, much more since the accident. "My running feels to have arisen from the break rather than something I'd had before. The small achievements I made with each session meant everything to me, no matter how incredibly small each step – literally - was. When I first tried running again five months after the crash the best I could do was to lurch along for five limping steps with teeth tightly clenched, then stop for a few minutes waiting for the agony to subside before I could have another go. I felt almost like I was learning to walk and run again from the very start, as a baby would, and that these were my very first steps. If I could get through this rehab and one day run again, I'd think as I power-lurched along, I could do anything. And compared to how I used to be before running and how my leg changed me, I think I can," Lisa says.

Her favourite experience involving running occurred when she and her partner Dan were travelling during this time. "We'd been down to Victoria for a quick trip away to buy a motorbike. Towing it home we stopped on the side of the road just south of the Queensland/NSW border, north of Bourke. This stretch of road is like driving on the moon, soft piles of grey sand on either side of the road and little scrub or vegetation. It was twilight when we stopped and in the dim light the lunar resemblance was even more striking. I was at the stage of my rehab in which I could walk without my walking stick but with a heavy limp. Hobbling around the soft sand stretching my legs, a light bulb flashed in my mind.

"I started running on the sand. It was so soft that my landings were gentle enough not to hurt my leg. As I lurched around cackling wildly I felt as Neil Armstrong might have when taking his first steps upon the moon. The feeling of running was incredible, though running might be too grand a term for what could better be described as a powerlurch. The elation I felt at getting as close as possible to my goal of running again was incredible and the vague notion of speed it gave me as I bounded around was intoxicating. I'll never forget that feeling. Something as a short jog that's so simple and readily available for able-bodied people was a reward long worked for and dreamt of for me and a little taste of my end goal of running again."

Slowly but surely Lisa has been able to return to running and enjoys it even more than before her accident. Lisa says she is a very competitive person. "When I started running I got a great feeling from beating my own little records along the way. The first time I ran 10km I phoned my partner while still warming down on the treadmill, absolutely elated. Earlier in my training I'd also done this when I'd first made 5km, 3km, and just 10 minutes of non-stop running. I love to see the improvements in my running and in my body with each session."

Lisa says the feeling of accomplishment has been much greater in her running than it ever was in her swimming. "Although I reached a high level in that sport, it was something I'd been doing since seven - whereas running was something I'd always found difficult, and was my new adult undertaking."

Running has been everything she imagined it would be. She loves the feelings of freedom, calmness and clarity it brings her. "I run for that feeling, the runner's high. The fact that my competitive spirit is also sated with each effort makes running holistically satisfying."

While Lisa loves swimming, she prefers running. "I don't get a swimmer's high with a good session. When I'm fit and strong it feels fantastic to pull myself through the water and meet tight time demands on a big set but I also still feel too attached to external factors to really get that relaxed, zoned-out high I get from running. In swimming I'm avoiding others, watching the clock, tumble-turning every half a minute. When I'm on a long run I just run and it's those long runs at a strong pace I prefer most of all. You can't even approximate a runner's high by doing a long swim, it just doesn't happen, there's no equivalent."

Making time for her training is something she has been used to since she was little and she simply does. "I'm reasonably guilty of fitting my life around running, rather than the other way around. I have a strong sporting background so changing my training to fit running in wasn't an issue. The difference is that running is much more important to me than those other sessions of gym, elliptical or swimming were. I get really cranky if I miss out."

Lisa's job as a paramedic in a very small town is a big challenge to her running as she has to stay within one-minute proximity of the ambulance. That means she cannot run outside if she is on call. "Being a small station we take the ambulances home and work overnight on an on-call basis, meaning that out of hours I'm not working as such but I still need to be available at a moment's notice should an emergency arise that I need to attend. There's no way I'm covering the second half of a 10km run outdoors in time to meet the one-minute response window required of work. For this reason I've bought a treadmill and do nearly all my running on that at home. Now my running is fitting into my partner's life more and more as it's a training tool he's able to use too for walking and running."

Lisa typically runs every other day in the afternoon and tends to be consistent. She also still swims and works out in the gym, with those sessions aimed at supporting her running. "I swim every morning. On non-running afternoons I try to use the elliptical at the gym which I find fantastic as a zero-impact running alternative."

When she has a day off work and is not on call, she uses the opportunity to run outdoors in the morning. She keeps track of her training, running and otherwise, in an online blog. The people close to Lisa are very supportive of her passion for running and she believes they understand what running means to her. "My partner used to run himself and can identify with the feeling of a great run and the sense of accomplishment that a good session or meeting a training goal can give. What he doesn't often understand though is why I train so much."

Lisa often trains twice a day including swimming and gym workouts. "I run once every two days so it makes up 25 percent of my training: but 100 percent of my training is with the intention of benefiting my running. Coming from a non-sporting background, two sessions a day is far more than my partner could imagine doing. For me it's normal and something I grew up with."

A great session leaves her feeling fantastic and satisfied. "And if I have also made some kind of PB or progress point I feel absolutely elated. I'm not above ringing people to boast before I've even warmed down. When I've made another step further along my training and performance plans I can't wait to write it down, put it into my blog, and I suppose mentally tick off that box inside my mind."

These days she is only disappointed with a run during which she struggles if she could have prevented it such as by drinking less alcohol the previous night or getting enough sleep. "I note how it makes me feel to have wasted a session, when a year ago with a broken leg I would have given my left arm to have had a sound leg to run on and would never have wasted that privilege. Beating myself up over a mistake won't help much, but I remember that feeling and try to recall it when I'm deciding between water and bed or another glass of that nice red."

Running always lifts Lisa's spirits. "Before the run I'm usually pretty excited and am looking forward to it. Afterwards I feel a kind of calm satisfaction and am much more relaxed. I usually run in the evening because of my leg – if it's cranky after a run I don't have to walk around on it all day. But when I do run in the morning I find I'm much more easygoing throughout the day. Things don't bother me as much, and I just feel generally more confident and capable."

Being a runner is very important to Lisa. "Running is a major part of my life, and increases its quality manyfold. It's a source of satisfaction and personal achievement that's always with me, no matter how other aspects of my life might be faring. It's a source of accomplishment dependent upon me alone: I have no one else to credit it to and nobody else to depend upon to make it happen – it's mine alone. Running is now my main exercise routine, whereas in the past swimming and Ironwoman training were. The health benefits are important to me, and I have found that of all the sports I have done there is nothing quite like running for its fat-melting qualities and aerobic capacity benefits."

Her athletic endeavours have always been a big part of Lisa's self-esteem and self-image. Running is as well. "Having done serious sporting training since I was seven in one form or another, being fit and having an athletic body is enormously important with regards to self-esteem and self-image. It's who I am – I'm a runner, I'm a swimmer. It defines me in both my looks and personality. I do feel better when I'm looking strong and fit, and not carrying too much on top, and at the same time I feel better inside because my fitness represents inner, as well as outer, strength to me. It is strength in character to pursue an activity that is often uncomfortable, that takes me away from the comforts of couch and cake, and that must be regularly attended despite the weather, mood or how busy I might be.

"I am proving to myself and to others time and again that if I have the strength and dedication to achieve that, then I can achieve anything."

Lisa believes that being a runner is a lifestyle and one that she expects to stick with for a long time. "Being a runner can't help being a lifestyle because it's easy to spend so much time doing, thinking about and planning your time around it. Generally though, you can't run if the rest of your lifestyle is wrong. It just doesn't fit in with eating poorly, drinking too much and burning the candle at both ends. Going out for the night is awesome fun, but no dance club or synthetic pleasure tops that of getting up early to run in cool early mist when the rest of the world is asleep and you're alone with your footsteps."

The single-most important thing about running for Lisa is that it allows her to completely focus on herself. "It's escaping from the world into something that's mine alone – my personal endeavour, my goals, and my achievements. In a world in which you're always contactable, that's always asking something of you, in which so much is governed of what you can do and when you can do it, running is the untouchable antidote."

CHAPTER 21
Thoughts of a serial marathon runner
"Running fits in as a matter of routine and as an unquestioned part of every day life."

Elizabeth Bennett loves running marathons. She has run more than 30, and counting. So far her fastest time for the 42.195-kilometre race is 2 hours and 59 minutes (plus 38 seconds) set at the Gold Coast marathon in July 2007. Two months earlier she had finished the Canberra marathon in 3 hours and 38 seconds which was a 9-minute improvement of her previous best time, impressive in all regards. She has won several races, breaking the tape at five marathons: Perth (2008), Alice Springs (2004 & 2005) and Hobart (2004 & 2009). "They have all felt different, depending on whether I've had to chase to get ahead and stay ahead or if I've been fading and had to hold off someone coming up to pass me. Neither scenario is comfortable. Essentially it really isn't over until the fat lady sings or the marathon equivalent: stepping over the finish line first. I had a few girls in front of me in the Perth marathon for quite a while. At 39km I took the lead. That made the win even sweeter. I really had to fight for it. When I went past the last girl at 39km, I knew that if she lifted I would unlikely be able to go with her. Fortunately she was spent and I ended up coming in 65 seconds in front of her. Whew," Elizabeth says.

Often the final kilometres of a marathon spark an individual struggle between following the determination of the mind to stay strong and the signals of the tiring body to slow down. This happens regardless of whether you're aiming for your personal time goal or whether you're competing for a top placing. "I've heard lots of people say they use mantras. I don't. Only because I can't really think of any that are convincing enough for long enough. I think I mostly just have conversations with myself, between my mind and body - with my body wanting to quit and my mind not letting it. When I'm in front and feel like I have nothing left and someone could pass me, I tend to oscillate between thinking, 'No way, not after all the hurt I've been through' on the one hand and 'If she gets in front then good luck to her, she deserves the win more than I do because I've got nothing left and obviously she's been able to drag something extra up from somewhere' on the other. That's about as simple and as sophisticated as it gets. To my mind that shows how instinctive or basic running for your life is," Elizabeth says.

Elizabeth took up running in 1984 at the age of 21 because her boyfriend at the time had done so. She was then focused on hockey and thought improved fitness would benefit her game as an A-grade player. But soon she ran for the sheer joy she felt doing it. "I quickly developed an intense love of running, particularly long-distance running, for its own sake. It didn't take long for running to equal my love of hockey and then surpass it. This was expedited by some serious hockey injuries including having my face and shin split open in separate accidents, a broken collarbone and knee surgery."

Besides a passion for hockey, which lasted 18 years, she has also been an enthusiastic and dedicated martial artist: a full-contact kick boxer. She trained and competed as a light-bantam weight and mini-fly weight. "Running has always been important in its own right and as part of my hockey and martial arts training. Running however has withstood the test of time, multiple injuries and several lots of surgery. I am still running but I am no longer playing hockey or kickboxing. Running is a holistic thing for me. I love it for the multi-dimensional enterprise it is."

Being a runner is crucial to Elizabeth. "It is who I am. Running fits in as a matter of routine and as an unquestioned part of every-day life. I don't question its priority and where it fits, and neither does anyone close to me. I refuse to miss runs for travel, work or any other reason. If other things don't fit around running then I don't do them. I've been a runner for so long I can't really remember not being a runner. I guess that adds credence to my view that running or being a runner is who I am," she says.

People close to her are supportive of her passion for running because they have to be, Elizabeth says. She says they understand what running means to her to the extent that she believes they can. "They are not me and don't relate to running themselves the way I do. They do their best to equate it to things they are passionate about and understand it from that point of view. And really, unless you feel it, that's the most you can expect from others in the way of support for your addiction to running."

After more than two decades of running, Elizabeth has learnt a lot about her body and mind. She feels satisfied, exhausted and happy after a great run. She has learnt to value those days when running doesn't feel that great. "I appreciate good runs because I have my share of crap runs and you don't get one without the other. A bad run reminds me of the value of humility and drives me to run better the next time."

What determines whether she feels it has been a great run or a bad one is a complex question, she says. "Sometimes it's about how I feel mentally and/or physically. Sometimes it's about running a particular route faster than before or going exploring and running an entirely new discovery route. Great can mean different things. I'm very in tune with my body and have been a long distance runner for many years. I still get a buzz after a good run which can last for hours or most of the day. But I recognise it for what it is and don't get lulled into thinking the world is great or the next run is going to be fantastic because of it. I enjoy the feeling, knowing that it is endorphin-produced and not a lasting reality in any sense."

Running always improves her mood, regardless of whether it was good or bad to start with. Elizabeth runs at least seven times a week, a regime that she has maintained for many years along with a full-time job and family consisting of a husband, two children and a dog. She follows a training program and keeps track of her training, logging distances, routes and comments about her runs in a diary.

"I am disciplined and like both variety and hard work. A training program provides that. I vary training sessions in consultation with my coach if I am over-fatigued or injured. I generally prefer to run alone. If I run with others I generally prefer to run with guys rather than girls, and guys who are better runners than me. The social aspect of running is not important to me at all. For me running is a solitary enterprise and I like it that way. I like talking to others about running but I don't see running training or racing as social events."

She has made new friends because of running, yet has also found other friendships adversely affected by her active lifestyle. "I have become distanced from those who judgementally accuse me of obsessing over running and who see that as a negative thing. I think that is their problem, not mine. I'm the first to admit I obsess over it. Some say I've become more obsessive but I think what they mean is that running is the demonstration of my obsessiveness and the extent to which it can go."

Elizabeth considers herself competitive when she runs. "But only against myself and my previous personal bests. I don't care what other people run." Neither does she care to recommend others to take up running. "I don't care if other people run or not. They should do what they want to do."

CHAPTER 22
My time reserved for running is sacred

"I have completed eight half marathons, two marathons and countless shorter events - I still struggle to call myself a runner."

Margot McGinness, 41, first laced up her running shoes about six years ago when the youngest of her two children began attending playschool. That gave her two child-free mornings a week. "I had always been very active but hadn't had too much free time with two young children. I started running because I wanted to regain my fitness after a few years at home with children. I needed to lose some weight and as I still didn't have huge chunks of available time to devote to a team sport with pre-determined practices and game times running was perfect. I could go when and where it suited me and for as long or as little as I liked. It also required little in the way of outlay for equipment and club fees."

These days Margot guards her time reserved for running closely because she has found that being a runner addresses other needs besides fitness and weight management. "It is definitely me-time and has expanded into girl-time too as I run with a small group of other time-poor mothers balancing work, family and fitness. So it now also fulfils a social purpose in my life."

Margot gave up playing competitive tennis because it annoyed her Achilles tendons and affected her running. She does strength training at the gym to improve her running, and adds triathlons to her schedule if it suits her run training. "Other activities have to fit around my running. Running is a very important part of my life. I love it. It keeps me healthy, fit, happy and sane – and that is good for my family."

She trains consistently because enjoys it. And even if a session on occasion doesn't go as she had hoped, she knows she will probably feel better in the next one. "When it is a great run I feel fantastic. There is no better feeling: it can keep your spirits buoyed for days and life is good, nothing bothers me. When it is a crap run or race, I feel very flat, disappointed and cranky but never disheartened - it motivates me to do better next time."

Typically Margot will train early to avoid unforeseen changes to her schedule preventing her from doing her workout. "I run four times a week when I am training for a specific event, three times a week if I am not following a program for an event. I am very consistent with my runs, otherwise I get very cranky. Usually I run very early in the morning so that life does not interfere with my running. Then I am set for the day and whatever it holds. This doesn't always play out so I make time somewhere else in the day for my run. It is generally not negotiable. I hate to miss runs. I get very edgy and do my best to squeeze something into the day I am supposed to run even if I have to compromise on the distance. Sometimes I feel guilty if I miss a session because I am feeling run down. I feel like I have to make it up sometimes. If I miss a run because life gets in the way I get grumpy and preoccupied with finding an opportunity to get out. The whole family has to wear the mood of me not being able to run."

While Margot may do her shorter, easy training sessions alone and listen to music on her iPod, she prefers to do her long runs and speed sessions with other runners. "It's good to know others are going through the same discomfort. There is an unspoken bond as we lap around the track or do one-kilometre repeats striving to take a few seconds of our previous laps. I usually run with other women which is just the way things have turned out. It serves a social purpose for us now too."

The social aspect is very important to her, partly because she used to play team sports. "I like the company of others in my sporting endeavours. My running friends are like a team to me. We often train for the same events, race together and sometimes travel away together, united in a common love of running."

Some sessions lend themselves for good heart-to-heart chats. "Anything and everything is open for discussion: children, husbands, school, work, family, news, religion, politics, travel, dogs - nothing is off-limits. Usually what is talked about on a run stays on the run. Not much talking is done on tempo runs or speed sessions though – just focusing on form and recovery. Constant chatter on long runs can be a little annoying sometimes.

"However we all seem to have an understanding that at times we zone in and out. Companionship is enough, talk is not needed."

She relishes spending time with her running friends. The non-running people close to her are not really supportive of her training, she says. "They just accept now that running is my thing, my passion. Most don't understand. They think I am crazy but they just know that is what I like to do. I don't think they truly understand what I get out of running and they definitely don't understand my continued commitment to it. As most of them don't run I don't expect that they would understand – only other runners can understand. I have always been a very driven person, determined and committed. If I wasn't into running it would be some other sport."

Margot usually follows a specific training program for key races, such as the three marathons she has run. "I usually use a program from some source for half marathon training and 10km. I find that using a program gives a focus to my training and takes the thinking about of each run, avoiding 'What will I do today?' I just look at the program and follow it. I am the sort of person who likes structure and routine and a program gives me that. It also reassures me I am on the right track to possibly achieve my goal."

Margot is committed to doing her training, motivated by her desire to run faster. "Generally I stick to my programs 100 percent. Only sickness or extreme family circumstances will cause me to miss a session. If I do miss a session I always try to make it up. I never skip a session just because I can't be bothered, even when I am tired. I make myself do it. I am a very competitive runner only in the sense that I am competitive with myself. Even at my age I am keen to get a bit faster and set a couple of new PBs each year. I relish the challenge - that is what keeps me running. I will never win anything in an event so the clock is my competitor, the thing I strive to beat each time. If I didn't race I wouldn't run so regularly or so zealously. Racing is what drives me - it is my motivator for training. Otherwise, what is the point? I think I would lose interest if I didn't race."

She particularly loves running because it makes her feel strong and very fit, Margot says.

"I feel proud of my efforts and commitment to training programs, so I feel good about myself, even if I don't look as good as I'd like to. Running clears my mind and keeps me sane. I hope to keep running for many years yet – so many races to do in many different states and countries. Running is kind of a lifestyle for me. It doesn't define me but it is very important to me."

CHAPTER 23
Running keeps my mind in check

"Any form of exercise has to be a lifestyle. It has to be woven into everyday life so that it becomes one of the things you just do."

Shelley Kirkwood became a runner about eight years ago when she was in her late 30s. After training on a treadmill for a while she joined a running club because she wanted to complete a half marathon. Her motivation to start running was fourfold: fitness, weight, health and social. These days she runs because she loves running. "Once you have run, the enjoyment factor, the endorphins and the challenge feature highly. Unless you have run, you don't have those physical and emotional impetuses to continue. The health benefits are still very important," she says.

Shelley runs four to five times a week consistently and follows a training program as it allows her to set goals and stay on track. She usually logs her training. "One of the running clubs that I belong to has a log book and I write out a schedule for myself every week with estimated mileage."

She doesn't always stick to her schedule. "I do skip sessions, usually because work has got in the way or my mood has got in the way. I try not to. I do feel guilty for skipping sessions. I know how good I will feel when it is over."

Occasionally she feels she needs a break from training, not so much physically but mentally. "It sometimes gets to a point where I have done quite a few weeks consistently and don't want to any more so I will have a few days off. It's not so much the activity but the thought that I have to be somewhere at a certain time. That constant having to do I find a little tiring."

Shelley also swims and lifts weights at the gym. She loves her strength training. "I can't really compare the running with weights as the latter gives me the strength and the running the endorphins. I enjoy weights especially with a personal trainer who will push you beyond your preconceived limits."

In running she appreciates the way she feels after the session. "You have pushed yourself up the hill, the sweat is pouring out, the sun is setting and you feel yuk. But when you are finished it is that feeling of, Wow I did it. Running means an ability to challenge myself. It allows me to switch off, to escape negative thoughts because when you are running up a hill it takes too much effort to do that, so thinking about anything other than that is non-existent. It's a chance to enjoy the fresh air."

Shelley has made new friends through her running, while there are other friends she doesn't see so often any more. "That's only because there is less time to meet up with people. However, you can always combine the running with the catching up."

While most of her friends are supportive and understanding of her passion for running, her family is not so much. "I am on my own, so don't have anyone really who is dependent upon me. Mum is the one who doesn't really get it. Close friends are supportive as most of them do exercise as well, so they are very like-minded. My life seems to fit around running and exercise. I am not obsessive. However, it is important to me to do the exercise so I will often put that as a priority, which others don't understand."

Shelley says she changed since she became a runner. "Inwardly I think that I have become more confident. I have probably become selfish in that I will put the exercise before a lot of other stuff - social stuff. Outwardly on a physical note, I am more toned, my resting heart rate is lower and my lung capacity has increased."

She loves the feeling of a session in which everything goes well. "Those endorphins kick in and it is great. The challenge that you have set yourself plus the training that you have put in, has paid off and it feels worth it."

Her body doesn't cooperate each time. "If it is a yuk run, physically you will feel horrible, often nauseous and dehydrated. When those symptoms subside the mental negativity kicks in. All that effort and what has it achieved? Those negative thoughts mull around: I don't want to train, I feel defeated, it's not worth it."

A great run for her is determined by both physical and mental aspects. "The mental high outweighs the physical soreness - the latter gets pushed to the back. On a bad run the mental and physical downers join for a combined low. The sore calves, which were probably sore after a good run, now feel 10 times worse."

A great run will lift Shelley's mood for at least a day. "In saying that, sometimes after a good run where I have pushed myself but still feel good, I will hit a downer a day after and feel unmotivated. I did ask a naturopath the other day about this and she said that the hormones go a bit all over the place which could then explain the bad mood."

If she is not happy with her run, she may skip the next session. "This depends on whatever else is happening in my life. A bad day at work - which may be triggered by a bad run - combined with the bad run tends to de-motivate me to run for a day or so. Then I get over that, out I go and it's the best thing that I could have done. The oxygen pumps through and my energy levels have increased."

Missing a few runs in a row makes it hard for Shelley to get back into it. "Mentally I am fine, physically it's a little difficult. It often surprises me how such little time away can decrease apparent fitness. I did read that there should not be three days between runs, even if the third day is only 20 minutes."

When she's in a good mood, there's no question she will run, she says. "In a bad mood I will often push myself because I know after the run I will feel better. And if I don't - well it beats moping. But I guess on the whole the good mood is easier to run with than the bad one."

Shelley feels better after a run 99 per cent of the time. "The endorphins certainly kick in. So physically and mentally I feel better. I may be tired or sore but still I will feel better."

Running has improved her quality of life. "I am healthier, so hopefully my immune system is stronger to combat those nasty bugs floating around. My energy levels are usually quite high. But I do have to go to bed early. I have difficulty with going out at night and staying awake. My heart, lungs and bones should be stronger. These combined I hope will allow me to lead a longer, more active life."

The health benefits of her running lifestyle are always on her mind. "They are probably my major motivation. But it does need to be combined with other exercise, such as weights and swimming and yoga. I do think that to only run puts too much stress on the body, plus it can be monotonous."

She is healthy because she runs, she says. "Because my heart and lungs are working well and because oxygen is moving around the system. To maintain a degree of fitness through running, nutrition intake must be at a sustainable level. Alcohol must be kept to a minimum. Sleep must be adequate. If all those elements are not at a healthy level it just won't work."

Running is important to her self-esteem and -image. "One of the reasons for me to run and to maintain fitness is to keep my weight under control and therefore to be healthy. Ideally this will translate to the outside by looking fit and strong. This in turn boosts my self-image. I like to look as good - healthy - as I can."

Shelley began running on the treadmill at home. She still likes to run alone at times but also appreciates training with others. "I enjoy the company of others on longer runs – it keeps me going. The downside is that relying on people can be a problem. I really need self-motivation. If someone joins that is great but if not, there won't be disappointment. I do enjoy group drill sessions. They are fun and can be inwardly competitive. I prefer mixed groups, especially with drill sessions."

Her running has become social as she joined two groups. "I quite like starting out with the group. If I fall behind and am on my own, that is OK, as we will all meet up at the end. I used to run with a close group of friends and that was great. We'd all stay around after the run, stretch, have water and a chat."

When she runs with a group she likes to be near the front. "This depends on how good they are and whether I am capable of staying near the front. If my fitness allows I do try to keep up towards the front. I prefer not to lag behind, not for any competitive reason but just so that I don't feel left out."

She finds it hard to talk during her training. "I am happy to stay behind and listen to others but I prefer not to talk. I can't do both, especially if lots of exertion is involved."

Shelley has suffered running injuries, typically calf problems in her case. "Having an injury has never made me feel like not running. It is something that I need to get better and then get back to my routine. Through an injury I have been able to do some other form of exercise so I am not completely idle."

She is competitive in the sense that she aims to better her performance. "I want to learn as much as I can, put that into practice and improve. I enter races but not to be better than someone, more so to give me a goal for training and a purpose."

She can be quite determined when it comes to achieving her goals such as during the Sydney half marathon in 2007 which she regards as her worst running experience. "I threw up over the finish line and felt disgusting for three days after."

Her best running experiences involve the simple pleasures of daily training: watching the sun rise over Sydney Harbour as she runs across the Harbour Bridge or hearing the Kookaburras as she runs around Cremorne Point without anyone else in sight.

Running has changed her life. "I have become more confident. It makes me feel good that I can achieve that goal, be it a 10km or a half marathon. A large part of the population does nothing so I am doing pretty OK. Striving to be healthy with exercise and nutrition also crosses over into work. I work hard consistently and I can do that because of my exercise activities."

Shelley expects to keep running as long as she is physically able to. "One of the clubs that I belong to has members in their 80s. Whilst they may not be capable of running all the time, they are out there walking, swimming and doing what is physically appropriate. They are inspirational. Also the exercise reflects in their attitude. They are interested, keen and social and I am sure that keeping to an exercise regime is instrumental to this."

Being a runner is a lifestyle. "Any form of exercise has to be a lifestyle. It can't be a fad. It has to be woven into the everyday life so that it becomes one of the things that you just do."

Even for all its physical benefits, Shelley finds the mental ones most important. "Running keeps my mind in check. It allows me to switch off and just concentrate on it, pushing any negative thoughts to the side and ideally out of the way. The focus becomes the activity, rather than what is mulling around in my head."

CHAPTER 24
Running has been a big hill to climb
"I wanted to be one of those fit-looking girls."

Shelley Maxwell-Smith, 33, had a clear goal when she took up running in 2006. Suffering from asthma, she had participated in very few sports until she decided to change that five years earlier. Shelley had started running and stuck with it for about six months, even finishing a 10km race, before a knee injury sidelined her. She didn't run again for four years. By then, Shelley was walking regularly in Sydney's Centennial Park in an effort to keep her weight under control. As she walked, she admired those who were running and resolved to try that again one day too. This time she enlisted the help of a running coach, Sean Williams.

Since then she has completed several 10km races and her first half marathon. What's more, with increased fitness and self-confidence in her athletic ability, she decided to add swimming and cycling to her training regimen and has finished several triathlons. Shelley credits running with changing her life. "Being asthmatic and totally un-sporty all my life, running has been a big hill to climb. Running has definitely improved my quality of life in a number of ways. It means I deal with stress more effectively for sure. I have made friends through running which is always a good thing. I feel better about myself generally and what I am able to do physically. I have better body image. I have learnt about my body. I enjoy Sydney so much more - running over the bridge or along the beach at sunrise is so beautiful. I have seen parts of Sydney and Australia I hadn't seen before," Shelley says.

As running became a part of her life, Shelley's lifestyle changed and she says it is much for the better. "It has become a part of my life, not an add-on to it. It has affected what time I get up in the morning, what I read, my friends, my conversation, my drinking habits - can't do a 20km run if you are dehydrated from too many beers, and my holidays with trips to the Gold Coast and to San Francisco to do running races there."

While Shelley has a demanding job, she makes her exercise a priority so that it fits into her busy life. She usually starts her day with a run, as she has found that is the best guarantee to get it done. "I make it fit. I like to run in the morning so that work and social things can't interfere too much. It doesn't so much fit any more - it's kind of become a part of my life. But it didn't always feel like that. Initially it was a chore. I had to get up much earlier than I was used to. Now 5:45am is normal. I sometimes like an evening run if I've had a bad day or feel the need to get rid of some crap."

As Shelley improved her fitness and health, she found that running also increased her overall sense of wellbeing. That payoff is a key motivator. Running has helped her to make better choices in other areas of her life which are beneficial to her health.

"Running is really important for my health. I'm lighter than I've been in years and feel stronger and fitter than ever. My resting heart rate has gone down and my muscle mass has gone up. I think about the health benefits a lot, they are an important part of why I continue to run. I think running is part of being healthy. I have reduced the amount I drink and try to eat healthily, which I think are also important to the overall picture of my health. The running is definitely part of, but not my sole reason for thinking I am healthy."

Working as a general counsel, she values the way running allows her to reflect and organise her thoughts, or to catch up with friends. Her spirits are usually lifted by a run. "It's some me-time. It's a chance to set goals and hopefully achieve them. It can be social, either at the running group or heading out with my girlfriends. It can make me feel strong and fit but also like having leaden legs and old, depending on the day. It's something I can feel good about, something positive I can do with my time. After a good run, it means a great mood for hours or on a few occasions even for days. A good run for me is either when I do a PB of some type, either in a race or in training. Or it's just a day when the run feels good, you are powering up hills, your legs feel light but strong, you could keep going for ages and ages. I feel strong and fit and alive."

She cherishes runs on her own but as her fitness increases Shelley also enjoys training with others. "Some runs I love to do with other people. I wouldn't push myself so hard if I didn't train with Sean's group for a start. Then there are social runs such as with my good friends where you get to have a chat, but I also know that they have pulled me along a few times. The time passes much quicker when you are chatting. I do love a good, long run on my own though - early Saturday mornings is a favourite for a two-hour session."

She's found that the social aspect of running plays a bigger role now that she is fitter. "It's not something I anticipated when I started running but it's becoming more important. For a long time I resisted running with others, probably it was partly fear of being too slow and partly enjoying the solitude of running. But now I like to run with others once or twice a week. For hard training, having competition is essential."

Shelley embraces competition and uses it to better her own times. "I am competitive when running but only with myself most of the time. So many people are so much quicker - I'm never going to be competitive at the front of a race. I do find myself being competitive in my training group with people of similar ability. When I started I was pretty much the slowest person there, now I'm probably about two-thirds of the way down the field. It's great to have people you know can beat you some days and try to chase them down. I am driven in my career but it's different to running. I was always pretty good academically, it came easily and I've been lucky to have had some great results and a great career. Career is easier for me than running at which I have no natural talent."

Overcoming the challenges of becoming a runner has lifted Shelley's self-esteem and changed her self-image. "It's massively important, not only because it helps my weight but my body changed shape too. The fact that I am now one of the girls in the park running around makes me feel good. Reaching goals is also really important to self-esteem. Hitting my 10km target and then finishing a half marathon later that year has been fantastic for self-esteem."

She had enlisted a running coach to avoid injury and bring focus to her training. With the help of her coach, Shelley achieved a dream goal in the Gold Coast 10km in July 2007. She had hoped to cover the distance in less than 50 minutes, which meant she had to run each kilometre in 5 minutes, or slightly quicker. "I hadn't thought I would do it until much later in the year. It was a huge surprise that I managed it so early. At 1km I was 4:50, which was great because it was a busy start. At 2km I was 9:40, at 3km 14:30. I couldn't believe it. Each kilometre I kept thinking, 'I can't do that again, I can't keep doing sub 5-minute kilometres'. I was trying to keep up with a group of guys in matching singlets. As the kilometres passed by they started to drop off. I was feeling great. It was a hot morning but I felt light and strong. It wasn't until I got to 8km in less than 40 minutes that I thought I might actually be able to do it. At about 9km you start to incline upwards but by then I really thought I could do it. I remember Eminem on my iPod singing, 'This opportunity comes once in a lifetime' and I was thinking, 'This is the first time in my life I could go sub-50 minutes'. I ended up with 49:23. I know it's nothing special for lots of runners but to me I might as well have broken the world record. It was an amazing feeling and I even smiled for the camera as I crossed the line. I haven't managed sub-50 since, although I've only done one 10km race since then. This year maybe I'll do sub-48."

With her fitness and confidence in her running ability improving, Shelley decided to prepare for a half marathon after about two years of consistent training. She was now running as many as six days a week. She finished the half marathon feeling strong. While she celebrated her accomplishment, she was already planning her next challenge: to complete a triathlon. Shelley bought a bike and enlisted a swim coach to improve her swimming technique with stroke correction classes. "I've always been an awful swimmer and my freestyle was non-existent. Now I'm trying to do two to three swims a week, two rides and three or four runs. I feel like I'm not running enough any more."

For her first triathlon Shelley chose a women's only event. She loved the experience and has since completed a mixed triathlon as well. While Shelley now trains consistently and has several running and triathlon races under her belt, she says that training doesn't necessarily become easier. Even when you are fit and getting fitter all the time, not every run feels effortless. Partly that is because the nature of some training runs such as speed or hill sessions, as well as long sessions, are meant to challenge your body because that is how you improve. Partly it is because your body may not feel that energetic every session.

On days when running doesn't feel so smooth, Shelley says, "It hurts. Your legs feel like lead, you're puffing like a train, you can't make it up Coogee Bay Road [a long and steep road in Sydney] without stopping. You wonder why you are out there at 6am in the pitch black and pouring rain running up hills that go on forever. I feel like a bit of a failure."

The determining factor for whether she feels she's having a good or a bad run is mostly physical, rather than mental. "I can get rid of mental stuff by running. Work out that problem, get rid of the stress. When you are a bit out of condition or are just having a bad day, it's all about the legs and the lungs for me. A bad run is when it hurts or it's a real struggle and I can usually feel that physically."

Yet no matter how difficult a run may have been, she'll always go for another one. "A bad run wouldn't stop me from doing the next run. Sometimes it will motivate me and ensures I will definitely do the next run. It depends how close I am to an event. If one is coming up and I'm feeling rubbish I'll probably push myself harder. Other times, I just put it down to a bad day and keep going as normal."

Shelley aims to be consistent with her running and sticks to her training program, especially after she found that missing a few weeks set her fitness back more than she anticipated. "I don't like missing too many sessions. I went back to the UK in August last year and ran a bit, but nothing like I would do here. I got back after just four weeks and my running had gone backwards by months. It took me almost three months to get back to my best times again. The first week or two were really hard, I couldn't even do the distance anymore - 15km had been easy before I left. I had to ease myself back into it by doing 5km, then 7km then 10km. Pathetic really. I don't think I will ever slack off so much for so long again, the journey was just too painful and I keep thinking how far ahead I would have been without the holiday regression."

Sometimes her mood influences her running. "I can have times when I am down and I lose my running mojo completely - right now is a good example. I have no motivation and getting out of bed is a struggle. But at other times a bad mood can really motivate me. I had a great run last week because I was angry and stressed and felt the need to kick the s**t out of something. Rather than my teddy bear or verbally abusing my work colleagues, I took it out on some hills, including my nemesis Coogee Bay Road. I felt so much better afterwards. I guess it depends whether I'm feeling down in the dumps or angry and stressed. Good moods don't really affect my running."

She sometimes skips training sessions and always feels guilty about doing so. "My main reasons are tiredness or soreness from training, the weather - usually when it is very wet - or sometimes just plain laziness and lack of running mojo. I skipped a Sean session this morning which I had planned on going to. I had laid out my gear, set my alarm and 5 minutes before it would have gone off, I turned over and switched if off. Instead of enjoying the extra hour in bed I felt guilty. Now I feel tired, sluggish and guilty. I hate missing sessions I have mentally committed myself to. I felt so bad I've just eaten carrot cake to make myself feel better - double whammy."

She does see differences in the way men and women approach running. "I think women are more competitive with themselves than with other people. They want to see what they can do, not whether they can go faster than their friend or colleague or next-door neighbour. I organised my workplace entry into the City to Surf this year. One of the guys who is a couple of years younger than me and much taller, knowing that I was a bit of a runner, told everyone that he would be devastated if I beat him, even though he hadn't done much training. This was only half said in jest. Needless to say I beat him quite comprehensively - by more than 10 minutes I think. Perhaps it's just my workplace but the guys are very competitive, whether they are playing squash, golf or running. It's all very good natured and they are all great friends but there is definitely competition."

Shelley has made many new friends through her training group and through meeting friends of friends who run. "Also, some of my existing friendships have gotten much deeper because of running too. I encouraged my friend Jen to join Sean's group last year. She was running a little but wanted to step it up. We did our first half marathon together in December and she's now a full-on runner. We are much better friends because of our joint love of running."

Besides her friend Jen she encouraged another friend Sarah to begin running. "Both started to get into running through me. I don't think I did that much. They saw I was enjoying it and also that I was looking fitter and healthier. I think that did the trick."

On the flipside, her non-running friends have had to take a backseat. "There are people I spend less time in the pub with. I haven't lost them but I spend more time with my 'healthy' friends and less time with my pub friends. There's still plenty of room for both."

Shelley likes celebrating her athletic achievements and rewards herself. "My treats are usually bad ones involving alcohol and food. I actually find that consistent training is its own reward, particularly when you are pulling PBs."

Sometimes a race doesn't go according to plan, which happened to Shelley in the City to Surf in August 2007. "My defining moment at the Gold Coast was only six weeks before. I had continued training, felt great and thought it would be a good day. I was aiming for close to 70 minutes, maybe even 70 or a touch below if I went really well. I had my red bib, the first pack, and was primed and ready to go. Then I had a complete stinker. At 3km I was on 5:00 pace but somehow at 4km I had lost a minute or two. It just got worse from there really. I had been training on Heartbreak Hill but I just couldn't get up it, or the next hill, or the one after that. I ended up walking parts of the course, very disappointed. My running mojo had left me at a most unfortunate moment. At 10km I was 55 with no hope of getting anywhere near a 70 finish. I ended up with an official time of 76, my watch said 75 but still very disappointing, event though I got back on the 5:00 horse for the last 4km. My reaction was to go straight to the pub. I had several drinks with my work friends before meeting up with other friends and carrying on. By the time I got home at 7pm, after about eight hours of drinking, 76 didn't seem so bad. Needless to say I didn't eat anything, didn't drink enough water and drank a thousand beers. Good work. You can imagine how I felt the next day, a disaster from start to finish."

The single-most important thing about running for Shelley is the way it makes her feel. "The endorphins are amazing. The stress and anger relief is second to none. The feeling of achieving a goal is the best. I'll probably keep running until I can't run any more."

Shelley began to run because she wanted to shed some pounds. "Ironically I now want to lose some weight to improve my running. My logic has come full circle. I run now because I love it - because I need it. If I don't run for a few days I feel tired, lethargic and sluggish. My calves get tight and I get jumpy legs in bed at night. I also need running to relief any stress. I do love the weekend long run, heading out on my own for two hours: just me, my music and some Endura - bliss."

CHAPTER 25
The power of friendship turned two women into marathoners

"When the alarm goes off I just have to get up and go whether I'm in a good or a bad mood because I know Stacey's waiting."

Karen Bradley and Stacey Harland live in Withcott, Queensland. These neighbours struck up a friendship about eight years ago and began meeting for morning walks. They also joined a gym together. In mid-2004 Stacey suggested they add running to their exercise routine. "I enjoyed the distance running events at primary and high school. I didn't ever win any races or break records but I got the odd second or third and represented my high school at the Darling Downs zone cross country. I had always been interested in doing a marathon and loved watching it on the Olympics but never really gave it much serious thought. I ran for exercise for a couple of years here and there, nothing ever too serious," Stacey says.

Karen, on the other hand, had zero interest in running. She liked their morning walks and resisted Stacey's suggestions to pick up the pace. "I've never been a runner – I didn't like it at all. When another friend did the 10-kilometre race at the Gold Coast in 2004, Stacey got all inspired and thought we should train to do the same thing the following year," Karen says.

Despite Karen's reluctance to try running, Stacey persisted. "She kept nagging me to. I resisted greatly, however she finally wore me down," Karen says. So Karen and Stacey began adding short stretches of running to their morning walks. "We started slow – just adding a bit of running to our walking, then a bit more running and a bit less walking," Stacey says.

Slowly but surely the two working mothers in their early 40s built up their running stamina. It wasn't long before they had a chance to test it. In early 2005, their gym organised a 5-kilometre fun run and breakfast. Stacey and Karen decided to participate. "We were a bit nervous and wondered if we could ever run that far as we hadn't done that distance before," Stacey says.

They finished the 5km race and loved the resulting feeling of accomplishment. The two women also noticed others runners doing that 5km stretch a second time. "We were totally amazed that some people turned around and ran it again. We were in awe. This helped us with our motivation. If they could so could we," Stacey says.

They had considered doing that 10km race their friend had finished the previous year at the Gold Coast, which had been the catalyst for their running. By following a training program the two friends achieved their goal and finished the Gold Coast Marathon 10km event in July 2005.

Finishing that first 10km within a year of becoming a runner at the age of 40 is still one of Karen's best running memories. "I was just on such a high from the whole race experience and in total awe that I had actually run 10km - and all with best friend Stacey of course."

The elation of achieving another goal immediately sparked ideas for the next challenge. "We were just so happy that we'd done the 10km. We high-fived after we crossed the finish and said, 'Next year the half'," Stacey says.

Both Karen and Stacey have busy lives, with jobs, partners and children. They have to make time to do their training which can be a challenge. But the mental and physical rewards they get from running motivate them to stick to the training programs they choose. They run four times a week, usually early in the morning.

"Sometimes it's a bit of a juggling act. On weekdays I usually get up at 5:30am for a run while everyone's still in bed and then I'm back home in time to get ready for work and kids to school. Sunday long runs can sometimes be difficult to fit in, depending on other weekend commitments, but the majority of the time I can manage to fit this in first thing Sunday mornings," Karen says.

While it may sound hectic, Karen finds the effort worthwhile because it allows her to focus on, and do something for, herself which in turn benefits her whole family. She says, "Running is me-time. Since I've had children I haven't really had much time on just me. I started running 3 1/2 years ago, and at times I feel guilty if I'm going on a long run, or going away for the weekend for a fun run - although that doesn't happen very often.

However, as the children get older it's getting easier. Running is something I can do. I don't have to be good at it but I can do it and when I want and how I want and I get such great benefits, both physically and emotionally, from it."

Stacey agrees. "I find time to fit running in around everything else. It is a chance for some me-time and a chance to have a chat with my buddy about all that goes on in our lives. The topic depends on what issues are pressing at the time. We find we can have a good talk while running. It is amazing how quickly you can get to the top of a hill while releasing all that anger. Otherwise we just chit-chat as we go. We are great friends and can talk to each other about pretty much anything."

And nothing is a bigger help to get up early when everyone else at home is still asleep than knowing that a running buddy is waiting for you. Karen says, "When the alarm goes off I just have to get up and go whether I'm in a good or a bad mood because I know Stacey's waiting to meet me. Which is a great thing because otherwise I know it would be way too easy to turn off the alarm, roll over and go back to sleep. I definitely wouldn't be where I am now with my running if I didn't have a running partner."

The early starts make them feel that they are getting more out of life. Stacey says, "We do often make the effort to look around as we are running – seeing the wildlife, listening to the birds in the pre-dawn light, looking at the views and watching the sun rise. We also think about all the extra hours of living we have had, being up and about rather than still asleep in bed."

Their new lifestyle has brought benefits to their health, and that of their family members. Stacey says, "I'm sure it has health benefits besides weight management. I know I'm a lot fitter than other girls my age in my touch team, plus all the other benefits that might not be obvious at this point in time such as reduced risks of osteoporosis, cancer and arthritis."

Karen says, "Running has a great affect on my quality of life. I have an interest now and it is such a positive and healthy one. I eat whatever I want - which probably isn't a good thing - but it's good to be able to not have worry constantly about what you eat. I feel well, fit and more confident with my body image. My running has had a positive impact on my family. My partner, being an ex-footballer, used to run from time to time but he is running quite frequently now and will probably enter some races this year. My children also sometimes want me to go on a run with them. Especially when it gets to school cross-country time they get very committed. I'm sure they would not be interested if it wasn't for my running, so that makes me feel great."

Stacey says, "My children will often ask me how far I ran when I get back all hot and sweaty. My son once said he wanted to be a runner just like mummy. My husband thinks it's good I get away for the odd weekend here and there to participate in a running event."

Both Karen and Stacey are now dedicated runners and have many other motivations to keep up their training regime. Karen says, "It is the great sense of achievement after a run, especially after doing a PB or finishing a race in your goal time; the extra time I get to spend with my best friend; the fat-burning and fitness benefits. It's a whole new exciting interest in my life."

Both women say they usually feel better after a run. After a great run, Karen says she feels elated, on a high and so glad she made the effort to do it.

Stacey says, "If we've just done a personal best for a time trial, or had a good speed session, you can't help but feel pleased with yourself. I also like the days when you feel you could just keep running – it's very motivating."

Stacey expects to keep running until they're no longer interested or no longer capable. "I don't know when that will be or which will be first. I do know that if Karen decided she didn't want to continue it would be a thousand times harder for me to keep running."

The single-most important thing about running to Stacey is testing herself. "I started running mainly for exercise and fitness but I want to see just how far I can run. I have goals I still want to achieve," Stacey says.

The two runners keep find newer and bigger challenges. As they pledged at their first 10km finish in July 2005, they returned to the Gold Coast in 2006 to run the half marathon. They did it again in 2007, and ran many other races in between.

In 2008, they decided it was time to up the ante yet again. They enlisted the help of running coach Pat Carroll in March and prepared for the Gold Coast marathon, held at the start of July. With their new program, they ran four times a week including one long run. Four weeks before race day they did their longest run ever which they clocked at 32.7km. Stacey says, "I felt strong and spritely the whole way and entertained the thought that maybe I could push myself for another 9.5km. So hopefully I have another day like that on July 6. Karen wasn't so lucky - she struggled the whole way from our first few hundred metres. But that too is a testament to her determination in that she kept going and going."

Those long runs come with a clear benefit. "Funny how anything shorter than three hours now seems easy. We have been talking and we feel we need another goal to focus on after the Gold Coast or else life will seem a little bit hollow. Though sleeping in for a couple of weeks will be nice," Stacey says.

Running has changed their lives. "If (when) we complete the marathon at the Gold Coast we'll be able to say 'If we can do that – we can do anything'. It has given us a can-do attitude," Stacey says.

Stacey and Karen did run their first marathon a few months later: as planned, they ran the entire 42 kilometres 195 metres side by side and crossed the finish line together. They ran their second one in July 2009, each setting a big PB.

CHAPTER 26
Reluctant start to running turns into lifestyle

"My partner used to ask me, 'When was your last run?' if I was a bit irritable. Too funny, he was usually right. I just need to go for a run."

Stacia Nelson was a reluctant runner when she started 11 years ago at the age of 19. She had just enrolled in a fitness leadership program at Mount Royal College in Calgary, Canada. "I had to take a cardiovascular course as part of the program. The instructor had us students go for runs once a week and I definitely was not a big fan of running at that time. Not long after I took a job at the local YWCA as a fitness consultant. My boss asked if I could help promote the upcoming fun run. Being new and wanting to please my new boss I said I would. I did not realise this entailed training members for the race," Stacia says.

She found out soon enough. Stacia trained together with the YWCA members for the race and surprised herself by enjoying everything about it. "We learned together, laughed together and crossed the finish line together."

Stacia kept at it. "I didn't have a choice when I started. Now running is a choice, it is a lifestyle for me. The same reasons I enjoyed it then are why I do now: for the social aspect, the sense of accomplishment, the feeling after a run and the melodic flight of running."

Stacia participates in many sports including downhill skiing, hiking, mountain biking, strength training and squash. She also teaches spinning classes. "I almost always prefer running to anything else. I say almost always because I prefer to run outside. And in winter it sometimes is not pleasurable to run outside due to the wind or ice. I live in an extremely windy area of the world. Running in that intense wind is dreadful. It's not peaceful at all and leaves the body feeling quite beat-up, as opposed to energised. And since I am not a treadmill fan, I would choose stationary cycling or squash to running. The only other time I pick something else over running is when the bears and cougars are out. I would then choose to go a slower pace so hike instead because of safety. The bear's instinct is to chase."

Stacia periodises her training. Simply put, this means she divides her overall training into periods that accomplish different goals. In her off-season she runs two days a week, keeping up her intensity and duration, and in training season she does four run sessions a week on average. Her work, teaching exercise science at a college, can be a challenge to her running. "Recently I burnt out on running because of my job. I had to run upwards of eight times per week. I have just come off a three-month break from running. I was injured and it was best to give my body a break at the recommendation from my health care provider. It feels great to get back running though."

Stacia, who is Canadian, moved to Australia for a while. There she followed a training program designed by Pat Carroll and kept track of her sessions. Back in Canada she still follows a training program which she regards crucial. "A good training program will ensure you progress appropriately, reducing the risk of overuse injuries and burnout."

While she tends to stick to her program, she does skip training sessions. "I have skipped because I have been sick, and then it is smart to skip, or because work needs to get done or I have company who does not run. Balance is important in life."

She used to feel guilty for missing sessions but now no longer does. "I have been running long enough that one session here and there is not going to bother me. Skipping a whole week is an issue though. And usually the headaches and irritable mood set in before the guilt does. My partner used to ask me, 'When was your last run?' if I was a bit irritable. Too funny, he was usually right. I just need to go for a run and all is well again. I don't usually have a hard time getting back into it. The only time I found running hard to get back into was when I moved from summer in Australia to winter in Canada: cold toes, burning lungs and throat, ears piercing with pain. Running was difficult then."

The sport is very important to Stacia. "Running in a way is how I take care of myself. It is my stress relief. It is my pick-me up. It is my time for me. It is a time to explore. I might be exploring the external environment such as a new town, country or park. I might be exploring the internal environment, meaning going through my thoughts and sorting them out, how my legs, back and breathing feel, and so on. I do notice that if work is going bad and I think about work when I run, my run gets really hard. It is amazing."

Being a runner is a lifestyle for Stacia and running fits into her life no matter what. "I am lucky in my job that I can make the time to run during work hours. It is part of my job to stay in shape. But when I travelled around Asia, Australia, New Zealand and Canada I would explore by running."

One of her favourite explorations was in Australia where she partook in a group tour. Waking up before anyone else one day at a camp site in Grampians National Park, she went for a solo run. "It was one of those spectacular mornings - Kookaburras, rosellas and other local fauna making their morning noises. I was running through the forest and came across the most stunning sites. The one that stuck with me the most was this large male kangaroo sunning himself in the middle of the trail. I stopped in my tracks. He just looked at me as I walked around him and continued running. I could have touched him, but thought better of it. I then ran to this waterfall and cooled off under it before I ran back to my campsite."

Back home in Canada running is the time she takes her dog out for exercise and socialises with colleagues and friends. "I have even been on a running date."

The people close to her are generally supportive of her passion for running. "My close friends definitely are. My colleagues run with me. My family is proud of me and now that I have been doing it for such a long time they accept it. They thought the long distances were a bit ridiculous. I find that if family things are going on I have to get up that much earlier to get my run in - they certainly would not change the schedule to accommodate my run. However I remember a couple of times when I have asked family to pick me up because I did not want to run back to the house into the wind. So I would run 10 miles one way and they would come get me."

Stacia has even found amazing support in unexpected ways. "A funny thing happened to me when I moved back from

Australia to my home town. I would head out for runs and I would be a few miles from my house or town and neighbours would stop to either visit or they'd stop me and ask if I needed a ride. Nowadays they are used to me being on the road and will offer me water. One set of neighbours takes extra effort to swath the grass on an old access road I run on. In spring the grass gets quite high so they cut it for me - about four miles."

She says that her friends and colleagues understand what running means to her. She is not sure if her family has always understood in the past. "They did not understand the distance I did or why I would spend money on a race entry fee. But despite their lack of understanding, they definitely accept it now."

Stacia has sessions in which she feels fantastic and others when she struggles. "When it's a great run, I feel on top of the world, energised, alive and that awesome tired. My philosophy with crap runs is that they are inevitable and it is best to get them over with before race day. Also a crap run is a great time to take notice of your training, eating habits, shoes and so on. It is a sign so listen to it, learn from it and move on. They are never fun but I am thankful for them. Running, as life, is all about perspective."

Both mental and physical factors determine if she feels it has been a great run or a bad one. "When I think about work when it is tough, my run gets harder. But I definitely have issues with running injuries. So when an IT band gets me and I have to stop it is definitely physical, but it affects me both physically and mentally. Tight hip flexors can cause me to stop as well."

A bad run doesn't prompt Stacia to skip sessions. "Unless the bad run is due to an injury but usually I extend a yoga session and my injury is taken care of. I am definitely motivated to run or train more but I am an exercise physiologist so I am smart about it. I am pretty understanding of myself and bad runs."

She always feels better after a run and will usually do her sessions regardless of her mood. "I just run. If I am sad I tend to sleep. I can say I run smarter when I am in a good mood. If I am upset, I run myself hard and then can't finish."

Running improves her quality of life. "I have more energy. I think clearer. I feel better about my body. I also am proud of my accomplishments through running. Running is extremely important to my physical, mental and emotional health. And while I say that running is social, I should clarify that I am not a social runner. I will run with others once a week but never more than that. It is my time for me and I need to be with me, myself and I. That is to help my mental health mostly."

While Stacia prefers to run alone she does have some great running friends she trains with. "They are like running alone with: we all put our music in and run in a group. We do talk but we usually save that for the coffee after."

The social aspect of running is generally not that important to her but it was when she lived overseas. "It helped me a lot when I moved to Australia. Joining Pat Carroll's group helped me find new running routes, meet new people and find more confidence in myself."

Running is extremely important to her self-esteem and self-image, Stacia says. "I am not sure it is healthy but to a certain extent I define myself through running. If I am not running I feel like I am doing a disservice to myself. A large part of self-esteem is looking after yourself - running is how I look after myself."

Stacia considers herself to be healthy because she runs. When she is running consistently she makes healthier food choices. She has also found it helps her combat the iron deficiency anemia she struggles with. "Despite doctors telling me to stop running so much, I find my symptoms are a lot better when I am running consistently."

She has recommended others to take up the sport. "Running has been such a gift to my life and I love to share my experiences in hope of inspiring others. I only try to convince those friends who have mentioned they should start to run. I definitely do not push it on anyone and want just to be supportive to those who are trying. I offer to take them for a run, help them with their technique and give them a program."

Running changed her life, Stacia says. "I enjoy mornings more. I appreciate nature and I certainly think that I have more confidence in myself. Running is my meditation - simple as that."

CHAPTER 27
Running has helped me cope with menopause
"At 54, I decided that I was not going to let preconceptions of age stop me and to return to the interests of my youth - one being running."

Susan Trodd, now in her mid 50s, began participating in sports during her schooldays, including in sprint races in athletics. In her early 20s she started running with the Hash Harriers in Hong Kong because she likes exercising in the outdoors. "After my stint with the Hong Kong Hash I stopped running for many, many years. Then a year ago at the age of 54 and after the usual trials and tribulations of life, I decided that I was not going to let preconceptions of age stop me and decided to return to the interests of my youth - one being running. That's how I met the lovely Susan Griffith at the beginners' jogging course which was a fantastic, well-paced, re-introduction to the jog," she says.

Susan loves the sport's low entry barriers and flexibility. "It's an easy sport to fit into your life as it's free, you can do it anywhere either alone or with someone or group," says Susan, who also walks, swims and does Bikram yoga. She plans to add cycling too. "My preference is probably running as I hit a zone where it's pleasurable. I love to sweat and push myself and, as said before, it's outdoors. I like to break it up with other forms of exercise."

Running means many things to Susan including: "freedom, exhilaration, health, happiness, camaraderie with like-minded people and pride in achievement - especially at my age." Susan aims to run two to three times a week but is not always consistent. She doesn't follow a training program. "Due to work commitments I know I won't stick to it," she says.

The people close to Susan are supportive of her passion for running. "Frankly it wouldn't matter if they weren't – I would still do it. There are some naysayers who suggest it may not be too good for me, being of a certain age."

Susan doubts the people close to her understand what running means to her. "I think only other runners really understand." Even so, her loved ones have noticed changes in

Susan since she resumed running, saying that she is fitter, has more energy and is more positive in her outlook.

The best running sessions leave Susan feeling like Charlie Brown's pet beagle Snoopy. "You know the drawing of Snoopy jumping up in the air, arms flung back, head back with the a smile stretching from ear to ear on his face - that's it. I enjoy the runs with a group which are at a consistently good, not overly slow or fast, pace for a good distance where I've felt we've all pushed ourselves and achieved something."

If she is not happy with her session she feels disappointed but doesn't dwell on it. "I usually just put it down to long work day, hormones, not enough rest or sleep and think it will be better next time."

When she skips a few sessions she misses the training and is motivated to resume it. "Depending on how much I've missed, it's hard to get back into. But I know that once I start I'll be so glad I did so that's usually the instigator for me to go."

Her mood does not affect her decision to train. "If I'm in a good mood I know running will just enhance it. If I'm in a bad mood I know I can run it off, although I may not be pleasant company for the people around me. It's not necessarily the mood that's the determining factor: it's the tiredness at the end of a long sitting-at-a-desk working day. Sometimes you just have to blank out your mind, just get those joggers on and go."

Running has had a positive affect on her health, both physically and mentally. "The health benefits are important. For peri- and menopausal women it can help alleviate mood swings and exercise is good for the calcium in your bones. Because running stirs up the endorphins and helps keep you fit and trim, it makes you more positive all around. Especially when you push through the initial stages, persevering and achieving your goals, you can't help but feel good about yourself which will then overflow into other areas of your life."

Susan likes to train with others, choosing it over solo training if possible. "I have always preferred running with a group and could never persevere when jogging by myself. I didn't start group running because of the social aspect but because I push myself more with others around. However, joggers are such a down-to-earth friendly bunch that you can't help but enjoy meeting them. I have improved with my solo jogs and am now pushing myself that bit further."

Susan has suffered an injury that stopped her from running temporarily and also thwarted her plan to participate in the 100km Oxfam Trailwalker. The experience left her much more cautious with building up her mileage. "I suffered from fractured sesamoids at the toe base early last year. I'm not really sure whether it was the running or the very long practice bush walks coming up to the Oxfam Trailwalker which I had to withdraw from. I had to stop all walking for exercise and running for eight weeks and would have been climbing the walls if I was allowed to. It made me more determined to get back into it again but also more aware of not pushing myself too hard too soon."

She likes to push herself to improve. "I don't compete against others, only against my personal best. I'm quite happy not to be keeping up with others, as long as I'm pacing myself to my best personal ability. I don't see myself as being competitive although I do think it important to try your best."

Susan hopes to keep running for years to come. She is inspired by a member of the Northside Running Group (NRG) she trains with who is in his mid 70s. "He is such an inspiration so I'm hoping for at least another 20 years."

Susan has made new friends because of running. While she hasn't lost any friendships because of her commitment to running, she sees some non-running friends less often than she used to.

She has recommended others to start running. "I've given the name of NRG to my nutritionist who has a lot of peri- and menopausal women as clients. She has seen how it has helped me. I strongly feel too many women give up when they reach a certain age, often more because of what society tells them."

One of her favourite running experiences is a tough speed session she did with her running group. "I thought I had run three circuits and had one more to go. Our coach said I had done my four - I must have just been so in the zone that I didn't even feel that last circuit."

CHAPTER 28
I became a runner when my walking buddies didn't turn up

"A good run can also just be about the conversation we have as we run. Sometimes I've had to stop because I was laughing so much."

Vicky Baxter-Wright began running about five years ago at the age of 40. Until then, she had been doing regular morning walks with a group. She and her walking friends met for their workouts near the meeting place of a running group. "One morning no walkers turned up but the runners were there so I joined in with them," Vicky says.

Her motivation to run was initially underpinned by a desire to stay fit and maintain her weight. "But it has become a lot more than that. I run to meet friends, take time out from a busy life, have time apart from family and work, and for an opportunity to challenge myself. In the early days I'd miss a run but now I hate missing a run."

She still walks, and also swims and goes to the gym. "Running is the absolute favourite. From a time-point of view I can get so much more out of a 30-minute run than a 30-minute walk. You can't talk when you are swimming. With the gym you rely on opening times, have to wait for your spot on the machines and are confronted with your mirror image wherever you look."

Vicky usually runs three to four times a week and up to five times if she is preparing for a race such as a half marathon. On Tuesdays and Thursdays she meets a group of friends to train with, which provides great motivation. "We never miss, unless we are away for work or holidays. I would never wake up on a Tuesday and think, 'Oh I can't be bothered,' and roll back over in bed. People are waiting for me and I would not let them down. On the weekend we'll do a longer, possibly more scenic run and I might fit in another run during the course of the week."

She logs her sessions when she trains for an event. "For my first half marathon I recorded everything: how far I ran and what I felt like. I'm not keeping a log at the moment but I will once I decide what events I want to do this year."

Vicky says she is surprised by how important running has become to her. "I've always maintained some degree of fitness, such as doing aerobics during the 80s, but the running has become a way of life. I look forward to the next session. My mood instantly rises after a phone call to girlfriends when we arrange a special run. I'm moody if anything interferes with my running schedule. It keeps me sane."

She fits running into her life by getting up early. "More aptly, how does my life fit into running? I am only half-joking. I am not an elite athlete of any kind. I am a 45-year-old woman with a family and busy job and life. My running times will never be of much note but that's not important to me. I run with girlfriends at 6am, every Tuesday and Thursday morning without fail and have done for years. I run early so that nothing can interfere with the run. I've learnt from experience that if you plan to run later in the day, things crop up and sometimes it just gets too hard. I run when the rest of the family is still in bed. On a weekend I run a bit later, maybe 7am, but this still allows me to run before I get involved in junior sport and other weekend activities."

The people close to her are supportive. "My husband was a bit bemused at the beginning. He is actually a very good runner who did sub-3-hour marathons in his time and he probably thought it was a passing phase for me. There have been odd times when he was a bit disgruntled that I was hopping out of bed, and out of his clutches, in the early mornings. But generally I think he's been very proud of me. I'm sure my teenage son is also proud of me. Sometimes we all run together in an event and I think it's great for kids to see their parents participating, rather than just as a taxi service. Close friends are supportive too and even work mates will ask how I'm going if I'm participating in an event. It goes without saying that all other runners are supportive."

She believes her family, friends and colleagues realise running has become an essential part of her life. "It's hard to explain to myself what running means to me let alone to anyone else but I think they know it's important to me."

Vicky has changed since she became a runner. "Physically I have trimmed down a bit but mentally it's been great too. I think

I've probably become less irritable but you might have to ask the rest of the family about that."

During a great run Vicky feels amazing. Such sessions boost her spirits for a long time. "When it's a great run it's just the best. It's great when you fly along. There is no huffing and puffing, or niggling knees or ankles, just a feeling like your body is working and in great condition. There is pure elation when you finish. The best natural high you can get especially if it's part of an event or something you have trained long and hard for. One great run can keep you going for ages. It doesn't have a use-by date."

Sometimes a session or a race feels like a struggle. "A crap run is hard. But I have never come back from a run and wished I had not gone. My aim is always to run and not walk. Even if it was a hard slog at the time I feel so much better physically and mentally than if I had just slobbed around at home. It makes me resolve to do better next time. Skipping sessions is not an option."

The factors that determine how she feels about her session are both physical and mental ones, she says. In a fantastic run she feels strong and powerful physically. She sets realistic goals and if she meets or surpasses them her mental attitude is positive. "A good run can also just be about the conversation we have as we run around the streets. Sometimes I've had to stop because I was laughing so much. How could that ever be a bad run?"

She is currently struggling physically with her training as she returned from a five-week holiday in which she only ran three times. "It was great to get back into it. Lovely to catch up with my running friends and they are so supportive and encouraging. Physically, it is hard to get back into it. No doubt I am running more slowly than before the break but I'll regain my fitness."

Vicky's frame of mind doesn't affect her decision to train. "I have a pretty fixed running schedule so my mood at the time isn't really important."

Running improves her quality of life and is also important to her physical and mental health. "I feel much more balanced. I feel physically fitter maintaining a healthy weight but also mentally stronger and more together. Running isn't the answer to all health problems. I still have all the usual health check-ups but I think it is an amazing health benefit. Running has kept me pretty trim which, rightly or wrongly, is important to me. I've never described myself as a runner. That seemed a bit presumptuous but I guess that if I have run three times a week for five years and completed three half marathons and numerous 10km events then maybe I am."

She has avoided injuries. "I have had the odd niggle but I have always been impatient to get it fixed and get back on track."

Vicky does most of her training together with her friends and prefers it that way. The social aspect of running is very important to her. "I love to run with my girlfriends. I run alone sometimes but group motivation is great. On runs we talk about everything: husbands, kids, TV and politics. Sometimes we laugh so much we have to stop. Sometimes we solve the problems of the world, all before 7am on a Tuesday morning. Mixed groups are also fine. I am not so good running with my husband as he can be a bit bossy and start telling me to run faster."

Vicky has made many new friends through running and lost one because of it. "When I made the transition from walking to running in the mornings I lost touch with my walking partner."

She has recommended running to others. "But not in a bullish sort of way. I don't want to come across as some tyrant or do-gooder. I'd invite them to join our running group and give endless encouragement and support just to start and see how they go. None of the runners I know would brag about their running."

Becoming a runner has changed her life, she says. "I think I am a nicer person. I get out my frustrations on a run and share stuff with friends before it becomes a major issue. Running doesn't mean one thing to me but many things: fitness, health, weight maintenance, me-time, de-stressor, friendships, achievement and some feeling of having control over my life. Maybe, if pushed, the most important thing would be feeling I have some degree of control over my life."

One of her best experiences involving running was completing her first half marathon. "I actually felt pretty overwhelmed by the whole experience and so unbelievably proud of myself."

CHAPTER 29
Running isn't important but the impact it has had on my life is

"They think I'm obsessed with this running drug. That I do too much, it influences my social life too much and takes too much time away from them. Bah humbug I say. They're usually in bed when I run."

Victoria, who only wants her first name published, started running at the age of 27 in February 2003. She had just begun a new job and found herself eating a lot of junk food three days into her contract. "I thought something has to give. Either I start doing exercise or I change my diet. I really wasn't up to both and I wasn't about to set myself up for failure," she says.

Victoria set about researching potential sports she could take up as an adult beginner. "After considering what my body shape might look like if I got into it, I decided on long distance running."

As someone who only walked as a last resort she decided that she needed help with becoming a runner. She paid a university student to meet her after work to train her. "After a month I did my first run with her - it lasted just under 30 seconds and I thought I was going to die. These days I consider anything under 10k not worth getting out of bed for."

Victoria ran her first marathon in 2007, supported by her running friends in Canberra. "My friend Marian did all my long runs with me and ran with me most of the last third of the marathon when it was getting very lonely and hot out there."

She sought guidance of a coach and followed his training program to prepare for her first marathon. These days Victoria aims to run five to six days a week but finds her routine typically allows for three midweek runs and a long run on Saturday. She gets up early to fit her training into her schedule. "I make running a priority. I get up early because that way it's done and usually I don't feel as motivated after work. If that means getting up at 4am then so be it."

Victoria skips training sessions, with reasons varying from tiredness to laziness to preferring a night out with friends to being injured. She says she definitely feels guilty for skipping sessions.

"But a balanced life is more important, so I get over the guilt pretty quickly," Victoria says.

When she skips a few runs in a row she misses it. "I feel like I'm in a funk without regular running in my life these days. It's hard to get back into it. I find it's easier to get back into it when I have friends to meet me and get me out there in the wee hours before work. Like good and bad running days, motivation ebbs and flows and I'm accepting of that. I'm more laidback about running than anything else in my life."

Victoria says she is not competitive when she runs. "I have enough areas in my life to stress me out without adding running to that list. I'm not so much competitive in other areas of my life, rather driven. I certainly push myself and am generally very focused on high achievement and personal success. With a half marathon PB of just under two hours, I'm definitely a back-of-the-pack plodder and that's cool. More time to enjoy the scenery and have a laugh. I noticed in a race last year that the fast starters all had very serious faces when they ran past. Those who had started in the slow pack with me mostly had smiles, and could laugh and talk with each other."

She has kept track of her runs in a log book, especially when she trained for her first marathon and if she feels she needs to keep her weight in check. "I give myself a two-kilogram window and when I reach that upper number, I concentrate on my diet and exercise diligently for a week or two to get it back down to the bottom of that two-kilogram range. That's much easier than trying to lose 5kg or 10kg or 20kg."

The desire to control her body weight is still her primary reason for running. She says she has a love-hate relationship with the sport. "I love that feeling I get around 15km, I guess it's the endorphins kicking in. I hate dragging myself out of bed before work, especially if it's dark. And I'll often whinge about the weather: too hot, too cold, too windy ... whatever. But then you'll get those perfect days, the weather's gorgeous, everyone's feeling great and no injuries in sight, and that 20km run feels easy, even though you're running up and down tough hills. And that makes it so worthwhile."

Since completing her first marathon she has added other types of exercise to her workout schedule. Her coach had her running 135km per week at the peak of her marathon training. Victoria needed a mental break from that rigorous routine. "I was feeling very over it all. So I started going to the gym and discovered pump."

She stuck with her gym classes for about a year, fitting them in with her running routine, as it made a positive change to her physique, she says. Recently she has swapped pump classes for rock climbing. Running is still her favourite. "Running, of all the exercise I do, is the one I love most. It's the best bang for your buck and you get time out to think or a great opportunity to chat with your friends if that's the mood you're in instead."

The people close to Victoria are supportive of her passion for running especially her partner. "After the marathon my supportive partner bought me a beautiful ring from Tiffany & Co and had it engraved with my finishing time - very cool. So now whenever I think 'I can't get up this hill' or 'I want to stop', I see it and am reminded that I completed all that training and ran a marathon and think I can run this little 15km easy."

Sometimes her training takes priority over her social life. "At times I've turned down social invitations because I have a run I want to do the next morning. But I try to have a more balanced approach these days - it's not the be all and end all - hence the plan for five to six runs a week and the reality often being only three or four," she says.

Victoria says the people close to her probably do not understand what running means to her and think she has changed since took it up. "They think I'm obsessed with this running drug. That I do too much, it influences my social life too much and takes too much time away from them. Bah humbug I say. They're usually in bed when I run."

Running has had a big impact on her quality of life. "It's the reason that I can walk up a steep hill or stairs and not notice. It's the reason I can try snowboarding or parkour or rock climbing for the first time and not suffer delayed onset muscle soreness the next few days. It's the reason I can eat as poorly as I do, and still get through a stressful day at work. And, really, it's the reason I can wear a slinky dress and feel confident about looking good, even if that dress isn't to your taste. So it's a total self-esteem booster. Running is hugely tied up with my self-esteem."

While Victoria says her health has benefited from her running by lowering her resting heart rate and boosting her overall fitness, she doesn't think about that much. "Mostly I think about how I can get away with those couple of beers on Friday night or that cake at morning tea or chocolate binge Sunday afternoon. It's all about the food."

She certainly doesn't consider herself to be healthy simply because she is a runner. "I'm not healthy. My diet is proof that I am not healthy. Some people think that because I run so much I should or I must eat well. What a joke."

Victoria likes to run alone but prefers to train with a few close friends. "And we don't even have to talk. Just being together is the best. The social aspect of running is significant. It's not just being social, but sharing that spectacular sunrise or having that support when you fall - literally.

"My running friends provide a companionship that no other friends can offer. They understand my need to run, and my need to not run on occasion too."

If she and her friends do talk during their training it is mostly light-hearted but it can also include serious topics. "The bonds I have developed with a couple of my running friends has meant they have been the first I have turned to when I needed to have that serious conversation and pour my heart out. And that means the world to me."

A great training session or race leaves Victoria feeling high and boosts her mood for at least a day. "I feel strong and healthy and happy to be with my friends. Depending on the distance and how chuffed I am, it can last to the next morning or the next run which is often the next morning anyway. Then it starts all over again."

A session in which she struggled leaves her feeling exhausted and drained, physically and mentally. But she will not let it affect her mood. "Perhaps when I first started out it might have put a damper on my day but now I realise you have good days and you have crap ones. A bad run would never stop me from running ever again. But a bad run also doesn't necessarily motivate me to train more. I'm not competitive with my running and I don't drive myself to run faster or longer in the same way I push myself in other areas of my life. I run so I can be more relaxed with what I eat, not to stress myself out about running well. And if you knew me you'd know I'm pretty carefree about what I eat."

Factors that determine whether she feels it has been a great or a bad run can be physical or mental. "Or worse - both. There are lots of influencing factors: my mood, the weather, whether or not I or my running buddies have any injuries, or a bra strap."

She's more likely to run in a good mood than in a bad one. "A bad mood, and dark chocolate and fatty goodness beckon."

Becoming a runner has changed her life, Victoria says. "I can do more things, like trying new sports and not suffer delayed onset muscle soreness. I've met some lovely people. I don't put on so much weight when I eat poorly for an extended period of time. I expect to keep running until I'm dead, mate. Until I'm dead. Well, you know, slight exaggeration but for a long time I hope."

She regards being a runner as a lifestyle. "Because it impacts on the rest of my life: the time I have to sleep; what I eat if I'm being careful and training; and whether I allow myself the time to do activities that put my running at risk. It's about priorities and I put running high up there. Not because running itself is important but the impact it has on the rest of my life is important to me."

She has recommended running to others. "I have managed to encourage and motivate non-running friends to have a go. I'm one of these people who always manage to do whatever it is they say they will. So if I've convinced them it's through my own actions. That's the easiest way. I guess you can't convince someone, of anything, if they're not open-minded."

For Victoria, the single-most important thing about running is freedom. "The choice to run or not run, because I can."

CHAPTER 30
Nothing beats the feeling of pulling on your running shoes

"I had decided I wanted to run until I was at least six months pregnant but my body had other ideas and I chose to listen to it."

Virginia O'Connor took up running in 1997 when she was in university and trying out for the police. "I knew it would be the simplest way to get the fitness required. I kept running as a good outlet. Then I was posted to the country and it became something I did every day," Virginia says.

While fitness is still an important motivator for her running today, enjoyment is the primary one. "I do triathlons as well as running but the run leg remains my favourite, probably because it is the one I do a bit easier then the others. Over the years I have substituted various sports and activities to replace running when I was injured but they have always been a poor substitute for the feeling you get from pulling on your shoes and heading out the door."

Family and friends understand what running means to Virginia and are supportive of her passion. "Because I've been running for 10 years it is just part of who I am. My family are used to that. They support me at races or competitions but also respect that it is my time. I have always tried to articulate what running means to me. It's not about being selfish with my time necessarily but about respecting what is important for my body and mind to function. Running has given me a healthy balance with life. It has definitely helped to reduce stress."

Virginia aims to run four times a week, though cuts back on run sessions during triathlon season to make time for swimming and cycling. She has kept logs of her training for specific races, which has both advantages and risks. "It increases the danger of becoming a little obsessive about a missed run or skipped session but it has the benefit of tracking injuries and diet, and their impact on your training."

Virginia simply makes time for her training. "Running is a priority for me because it is about my mental health as well as physical health. To me running means an escape from the real world. Nothing else really matters when you're out for a run and it's something I never need to think about - it just happens. Regardless of what else has happened or is going to happen that day, my legs will normally just roll themselves over and my brain can shift out of gear."

Virginia never lets her mood affect her decision to run. "I definitely find that running if I'm in a foul mood helps to lift that mood. I'll always come home that bit more positive after a run. I always feel better after a run. Some days it may be hard to get going but it's always worth it. Running definitely adds to my quality of life. It is an enjoyable experience that generally only has positive benefits. The single-most important thing about running is that it is enjoyable. The day it stops being fun is the day I give it away."

Virginia says the biggest change after she became a runner was her social life. "Becoming a runner opened up a whole new social circle. I have made friends with people who I would never have met if I hadn't joined a running group. Some friendships have become harder to maintain because of training routines. I guess some friends haven't really understood why I won't go out or have drinks some evenings if I have a big training session or race coming up. I've recommended friends to start running. I generally just use the good examples I have of its positive benefits to help convince them. In the end they will only take it up if it suits them.

"The social aspect of running is very important. Meeting for breakfast after a long run in Brisbane is one of the best things to do with Sunday mornings. There are some days when I prefer to do my long run by myself and others when it is with a group: you're talking for an hour and suddenly the run is over before you even know it. It doesn't bother me if the group is a group of girls or a mixed group, they each have some advantages. I do like to do my speed sessions with a group and a coach as it is so much more motivating."

Virginia is consistent with her training and follows a program to avoid overtraining and overuse injuries. "I hate missing a few runs. If I'm travelling I always have a pair of shoes packed and try to fit a run in. I skip training sessions when I have to. Unfortunately it is necessary to skip them every now and then. One of the most valuable things that I was told was that once a training session has been skipped it is gone. You can't go and make it up, so you just let it go past without too much concern. I feel guilty for skipping sessions so I try to make sure it's a good reason to skip it, i.e. family or work commitments and not because I was feeling slack. Although some days it's best just to listen to your body and stay in bed. I generally find after sickness or a break that I can't wait to get back into running. Currently being at the very end of pregnancy I can't wait to get my shoes on and go for a run."

Five months into her pregnancy Virginia took a break from running because of her physiotherapist's advice rather than her doctor's. "My doctor let me be the judge of my running and advised just to watch my heart rate and core temperature. I was guided by my physio to prevent injuries and instability which would prevent returning to running. When I fell pregnant I was training pretty hard: my long-distance runs were around 20km and I was doing two speed sessions a week. I dropped the intensity of the speed sessions immediately and then gave them away at about four months into my pregnancy. I didn't want my heart rate or core temperature getting too high. I had miscarried five months before, so I was extra cautious about putting the pregnancy at risk. I kept running distances of about 10km but at a very low heart rate and with a heart rate monitor on.

"I gave this away around five months into the pregnancy on advice from my physio as old running injuries were playing up. I am one of the not-so-fortunate runners who have had stress fractures. The first was in my foot and required a walking cast for a month. The second was right through my femur and put me out of running for months. At the time it was so painful I thought I'd never get back to running. I was so angry as it was something that I had caused by not being sensible and overtraining. Not running for that period of time made me just want to get back to it. I had to start with water running and cycling on flat roads and slowly it came good. Now it seems like a distant memory and I have learnt the hard way that overtraining is far worse then under-training," Virginia says.

While Virginia gave up running five months into her pregnancy, she has kept up walking on a treadmill at home, as well as cycling on a stationary bike and swimming which all allow her to control dangers and temperature. "Most of my girlfriends said they were guided by listening to their own bodies and this is the best advice I was given. I had decided I wanted to run until I was at least six months pregnant but my body had other ideas and I chose to listen to it. I just told myself it would make my return to running a bit easier and I didn't want to injure myself or the baby. I have been so lucky and have had an uneventful pregnancy. I think that my fitness, which was at least partially attributable to running, has helped so much. Keeping fit has allowed me to keep feeling OK about myself and not struggle too much with increasing weight."

Virginia hopes to resume running shortly. "I expect to be able to return pretty soon after having the baby. I have kept pretty fit and as soon as my body feels right and I have the doctor's OK, I plan to get back to running. The hard part will be that after a bit of a break I can't expect to be back where I left off. But in saying that, it will be such a pleasure just to be out there that I don't think I'll mind and with the addition of a running buggy I will have some good company."

CHAPTER 31
Running is a habit and I need it to feel positive
"I feel it's what the human body has been designed for."

Marrying a runner can have dire consequences, as Aimee Barrett's husband found out. "I have dragged my husband through two marathons with me," Aimee says.

Weight control and stress relief were Aimee's main reasons to start running when she attended high school in the 1990s. Now 28 and a physiotherapist, she runs consistently five times a week. "Running is a habit and I need it to feel positive. I enjoy the routine and the feeling you get from running - it really boosts my self-esteem and I get more energy from it. I love to feel fit and we now do a lot of outdoor activities in our spare time, especially multi-day hiking and altitude stuff thanks to our running fitness."

Her passion for running has shaped Aimee's social life, as she gained many friends whom she met because of a common interest. "[Non-running] friends think we are mad and obsessive but I now have many running friends."

Running to Aimee means freedom and friendships. "I feel it's what the human body has been designed for. I also swim but feel it can be a really lonely sport, while running with running clubs has allowed me to meet people from a whole range of ages and backgrounds. You meet people that you otherwise wouldn't."

Even so, she does often enjoy quiet runs, partly because it avoids the temptation of racing training partners when she shouldn't. "Often I like running alone or with my husband only. With friends and groups I find I can't help but get competitive which is great for training and times but not always what you need. I push the pace unfortunately. I love to be one of the boys and I am harder on myself than anyone else is on me."

Being a runner is a lifestyle, she says. Aimee plans to keep running as long as she can, which she hopes is for the rest of her life. Aimee has just spent 18 months travelling, which made sticking to her running routine tough and forced her to be creative. "Even though we were very active I really missed the running, particularly at the start. When possible we still went for a jog, even in Africa and the Americas. Also, most of our marathon training we did while on holidays in Croatia and France. If you are training for something, you just have to make time."

Running is very important to Aimee's self-esteem and self-image. She is conscious of the health benefits resulting from being a runner and considers her running routine one of the reasons for her being healthy.

Aimee feels better after a run than before because it helps her relax. When she has had a great run, Aimee feels a "huge high" and it will boost her mood for at least a day. On days when she struggles with her session, she slows down. She never skips training unless she is sick. At times that has been detrimental. "I usually run even when I shouldn't as well. I have had a lot of overuse injuries and it's so frustrating. I still like being outside. If I feel crap I just stop and walk and enjoy being outside."

Aimee considers herself a competitive person, whether it is running or otherwise. "Absolutely and in everything, but I feel competitive against myself more than others really."

She has recommended others to take up running and often offers to take those interested for a few runs. "I go for a slow jog with them a few times and see how they go. I am a very motivated person and am constantly surprised how much motivation others require when I can motivate myself easily."

CHAPTER 32
A great run makes me feel invincible

"I have more energy, am more motivated to take risks, I feel like I can do whatever I set my sights on given the right preparation."

Anne Marie Halton ran her first 5-kilometre race in 35 minutes in Noosa in 2000 without training. "A much fitter friend suggested I complete a fun run with her. I promptly fainted at the finish line and again when we went for brekkie."

Despite the fainting Anne Marie enjoyed the experience enough to start training, especially because running suited her schedule. She now prefers running over other forms of exercise because of its efficiency, convenience and the impact on her mental and physical wellbeing. "Initially running appealed because it fitted into a busy life. Now I enjoy both the social aspect and the meditative element when on a solo run. Running to me means fitness and important headspace. I squeeze running in between work, kids - I'm a single parent, partner and friends. But it has become a priority for me, almost like part of my identity," Anne Marie says.

A lot has changed since that 5km made Anne Marie faint. She ran her first marathon in 2007 which was a great experience. "Running down the finishers' chute at the Gold Coast marathon, the race announcer calling my name and high-fiving anybody and everybody like they were all there to cheer me on – what a rush."

The people close to Anne Marie are very supportive of her passion for running, and she believes they understand what running means to her. Anne Marie runs about three times per week consistently unless she's injured. She keeps track of her runs with a few notes on a spreadsheet.

A good run lifts her mood. "When it's a great run I feel invincible; faster, fitter, stronger and more Zen. I feel better all day and more motivated for the next run and to aim higher."

If her run doesn't feel that smooth it doesn't bother her. "I'm usually pretty content to have even made it out the door. When it's a crap run, I feel every one of my 45 years."

She feels better after a run. If she is in a bad mood she is extra keen to do her training. "I definitely feel the desire to run more when I'm in a bad mood."

Running has improved her quality of life, her self-esteem and her self-image. She also considers herself to be healthy because she runs. "It contributes to a much healthier lifestyle. I'm not often up for late nights or drinks with friends as I prefer early morning runs. It's the old cliché: running makes me a much nicer person, plus it increases my energy. I also like having a goal on the horizon. I have learned about myself, about focus and mental strength. It has been great: I feel mentally stronger and more resilient."

Anne Marie has gained many new friends through running, especially because of her marathon training with the Pat Carroll Running Group. "If you go through a challenging event like training for a marathon, you create a bond with others who have experienced that. The social aspect of running is a great motivator. I'd never have had the courage or perseverance to train for a marathon without PCRG support. It's a great excuse to catch up with girlfriends. When training for the marathon it was a fantastic opportunity for me to catch up with a close girlfriend. We regarded it as therapy and it made us much closer. We miss it now that she's pregnant."

She is on a training program in her race season and runs without one in her off-season. "In the four months before a race I like to tick off the training accomplished as one more step towards my goal."

While she will be flexible about the timing of her training sessions, she rarely misses any. If she does skip a session she feels guilty. "I often have to swap around when life becomes too busy. I only really miss sessions completely when injured or fatigued," Anne Marie says.

She's had injuries to her lower back and Achilles because of running that forced her to stop running for a while. "It's very hard to be patient and not run at all, as I hate the sensation that all the hard-won fitness and strength is ebbing away, but it makes me more determined to recover. Having a goal helps a lot."

Anne Marie competes in running races for the personal challenge and fun. She doesn't consider herself competitive. "I'm a middle-aged mum doing it for pleasure, fitness and personal challenge - there may be a bit of ego in there too. Though I do like it when I catch someone I had thought was faster than me."

She believes women approach running in a different way than men do. "In my experience men, especially non-runners, have an inflated opinion of their ability. Men are more competitive."

Becoming a runner has changed her life. "I have more energy, am more motivated to take risks, I feel like I can do whatever I set my sights on given the right preparation. I really admire those tough old women runners. I hope I'm like that when I'm 70."

The sense of achievement is the single-most important thing about running for Anne Marie: "Both in a day-to-day sense of completing a training session and in the larger sense of realising a goal by completing a marathon or running a PB."

CHAPTER 33
My life feels poorer when I do not run
"Nothing quite equals the good feelings and the lift to my spirit I get from running."

Anne Jones has been running half her life. Now 54, Anne started in 1980 after the gym banned her because she had lost too much weight by attending 14 aerobics classes a week. While she turned to running to keep her weight low, she credits the sport with helping her restore her health. "When I started running I was anorexic but to run better I had to get healthy so I had to change my diet and lifestyle. Running was becoming popular and the idea appealed to me. I didn't realise at the time I began running how enjoyable it was or that you could join clubs and run in races. I still run for weight control but also now for the health benefits, both mental and physical, and for the social outlet of running with other people. I also run for the sheer physical pleasure of it and the sense of freedom I get when running well."

These days Anne also does group fitness classes at the gym, like body combat or body pump. She turns to yoga or Pilates for injury prevention or rehabilitation. "Running is my favourite exercise. Nothing quite equals the good feelings and the lift to my spirit that I get from running," Anne says.

Becoming a runner has helped her to set and achieve goals in several areas of her life. It has increased her confidence and mental focus. "Running is one of the most important things in my life, probably pretty close to the most important. It means freedom, enjoyment, being able to eat, having fun, achievement, spirituality, being in the outdoors with nature, being healthy, being active and youthful and much more that I can't explain. Running gives me a goal to work towards and things to achieve. It gives me something to plan. It gets me out of bed in the morning. It's beneficial to my health as well. It's also beneficial socially. All in all, running has a good effect on my quality of life. My life feels poorer when I don't run."

Anne runs five days a week. Four of those are runs of about 30 minutes with a longer session of about an hour on the weekend. She usually trains in the morning. "I'm pretty consistent barring injury. On the days that I don't run, I do a 30-minute walk. I wish I had more time on weekday mornings to run and more time to get to the gym. Otherwise, it fits in quite well as I run before work. I find it best to run in the morning, so that competing work and social duties don't get in the way."

Since Anne began running she has become physically and mentally stronger. Especially those days when she has good training sessions or races are cherished experiences. "When it's a great run I feel fantastic, happy, pleased with myself, strong and healthy. It's a good run if I do what I have set out to do, in terms of distance or hills or speed, and I feel OK while doing it," she says, adding that she always feels better after a run.

Anne says that her run training has contributed significantly to her wellbeing. "Running is very important for my health - it lowers blood pressure, controls weight, lowers cholesterol, is good for your bones and helps with stress and depression. I think about the health benefits a lot."

Her mental state is also affected by her running, she says. "Running is very important to my self-esteem. It helps me feel good about myself. Now that I'm older I don't talk about my running and exercise so much for fear of ridicule from other people and comments like, 'You're a bit old for that, aren't you?' I only talk about it to other runners around my age. The self-esteem side of it is an internal thing that I keep to myself but it still helps me feel good."

Anne says she is familiar with most of the old wives' tales about running for women. "I've heard all sorts of strange comments about why women shouldn't run like it makes you sweat; it makes your boobs sag; you won't be able to have babies, and so on. There are lots of naysayers who will discourage women, especially women who don't fit the young and beautiful image, from doing anything for themselves. They also like to keep women in their place, usually at home looking after them. I'm sure there are lots of women who've been discouraged by partners, family and friends from running, usually for their own selfish reasons. It can be hard enough to get started, without having to deal with that sort of thing."

Anne says that it can be difficult to find support from family or a partner and believes her family and friends don't understand what running means to her. "I've generally found in the past that partners aren't supportive. My parents never really understood why I ran or why I did any of the things I did. Most of my friends are also runners or do other sports, so they understand, but I wish they were more supportive about injuries," she says.

She says her passion for running may have scared off possible partners or friends. "I have probably lost potential partners or friends because I have curtailed my social life to accommodate running."

Anne doesn't follow a training program as she has found it impossible to stick to one. She keeps a log of her training in a diary, as well as of her race times. She mixes up her runs, sometimes training alone and other times with friends. "I think you definitely need to do some of your training alone, as you're more aware then of [potential] injuries and other physical indicators and can concentrate better. Also, it can be good preparation for long races where you could be by yourself for quite some time. I prefer to run in a mixed group. I enjoy the male company. I like to talk while running, on any subject, serious or light-hearted. I have met people who don't like to talk at all while running and found it a bit strange."

Being a runner is a lifestyle, Anne says. "You plan the rest of your life around it: eat right, rest, do other helpful sorts of exercise, socialise with other runners, read about running, etc. I hope to run for as long as I can - at least another 25 years. This, again, is something I don't mention to too many people except other runners. I'm determined, despite health challenges, to keep running or at least to keep as active as I possibly can. I'd rather be active and die a bit sooner, than be inactive and linger on not being able to do anything."

She has made new friends over the years because of running. "I've met people through running that I never would have crossed paths with otherwise. Unfortunately, being sidelined with injury so much lately has interrupted the social side of running for me. The social aspect of running isn't as important as it used to be."

Anne will advocate running, but only after someone has shown an interest in taking up the sport. "I tell them about the running clubs here in Perth and how enjoyable that aspect of running is. I always emphasise starting slowly and building up gradually and tell people that walking is also very good exercise if running doesn't appeal."

Anne's best running memory is of doing her first marathon. "I wish I could run one again."

Recently it has been hard for her to train with others because she has struggled with injuries and stress-induced fatigue. "I've had injuries that have forced me to stop running. I am always determined to get back to running again after an injury. I try to work out the cause of the injury and how to prevent it happening again. I hate not being able to run."

CHAPTER 34
Planning my week ahead ensures my training fits
"The realisation that slower runners are still real runners is one of my best experiences involving running."

Caroline, who only wants her first name published, is 35 and began running two-and-a-half years ago, initially to lose weight and improve fitness. Along the way she has discovered more motivators. "While I still use running as a tool to assist with weight management and fitness, my reasons for running have shifted substantially. I now run for a variety of other reasons too. The main reason I run is because it makes me feel good. I live near the beach and love getting outside and watching the water. I actually quite like running in the winter when the seas are dark, the waves are crashing and there is light rain. I run to keep improving myself and my times. I also am involved with a running group so it is social as well," she says.

Caroline runs four times a week consistently barring injury or sickness. She makes room for her training sessions by planning ahead. "I usually pre-schedule my runs at the beginning of each week to ensure they get done and fit in with my work. I usually run in the mornings, before work so that it doesn't interfere too much with other parts of my life and my social life."

Like all runners Caroline loves those training sessions when everything seems effortless. "You get that fantastic feeling that you are running quite fast – for me, a floating feeling and it feels really easy like you could keep going for hours. And afterwards you feel like you are on a high."

She also experiences those days when running just feels hard. "Although some runs do feel fantastic, I don't always feel great during the run. Sometimes you really have to push yourself just to finish the run, like when you first started and every run was a challenge."

Determining whether she experiences a session as a great run or a bad one are typically more physical factors than mental aspects for Caroline. "The release of endorphins is definitely a sign of a great run. Although there is the odd run which has felt physically hard and mentally you have stuck it out to complete the run or maintain the purpose of the run. Then afterwards there is a great sense of achievement."

A good run usually puts her in a good mood for an entire day, she says. A session that felt hard doesn't ruin her day. "Fortunately really bad runs don't occur too often. If I have a couple of bad runs in a row I can get discouraged. However, it is usually a sign that I need to back off and have an easy couple of runs or have an easier week. Once I do that I am usually back on track again."

She only skips sessions when she is ill. She doesn't find it hard to resume training afterwards. "Occasionally I will miss a session because I can't be motivated. If I skip one session occasionally for a genuine reason such as sickness, I don't feel guilty. If I skip a session due to the blahs, then I do feel guilty."

Caroline doesn't let her mood interfere with her training, as she always feels better after a run. "I am definitely more motivated to run when I am in a good mood. However, experience has taught me that getting out there and running when in a bad mood can be very therapeutic. Running is a great way of mulling over problems and coming up with solutions or getting some perspective."

Running has improved her quality of life. "I have lots of energy. It positively affects my mood. I definitely feel more positive about life when running regularly."

While she considers running a healthy activity, she doesn't consider herself to be healthy because she runs. "Obviously running has a lot of health benefits. However, I am at the upper end of my healthy weight range and know my diet could be improved."

She likes running alone as well as with others. "Solo running is great for sorting out problems, thinking about things or planning. Long runs are definitely more enjoyable with a group. The social aspect of running is very important. Our running group participates in lots of fun runs and weekends away. We also do lots of other non-running social events. I have met lots of great people and made some really good friends through running."

She generally follows a training program. "Initially the programs were designed to ensure I can make it to the end of the run in one piece. I am currently returning from injury, so I am following a program to slowly build up the kilometres again. Once I have my aerobic base back I would like to improve my 10km and half marathon times. While I love getting out there and running, I find I am more motivated when I have a goal to aim for. For my last half marathon I enlisted the help of Pat Carroll online and improved my half marathon time enormously."

Caroline has struggled with plantar fasciitis, a painful foot condition. "Being unable to run has greatly improved my motivation. However it has been tough restarting again at a lower level of fitness. Unfortunately I didn't have the commitment to do water running."

Races are an important part of running for Caroline. "I am definitely competitive with myself when I run. I don't really care how I compare to my running buddies. In a fun run I definitely try to pick off runners throughout the race. I am not really a very competitive person in other areas of my life. Running has actually taught me a lot about setting goals. It has also taught me that by consistently picking away at something, improvements can slowly be made. I really enjoy races. These motivate me to train."

Caroline keeps a brief log of her training. "They are in my diary as the length of time that I ran. In the lead-up to big events, I may do some speed work and log these times."

The people close to her are supportive of her passion for running. She doesn't think they really understand what running means to her. "They think I am a bit mad. They are also convinced it is bad for your knees etc. They think I am this super-fit person. I am only a moderately fit runner."

While she hasn't lost friends because of running, she says she has probably moved away from old social circles which tend to drink and party heavily. Becoming a runner changed her life. "Running has made me become a lot more positive and a lot more health-conscious. It has also exposed me to lots of other like-minded people."

Caroline believes women approach running in a different way than men do. "I think men are on average more competitive about running. Many women are happy to participate and enjoy the health and social benefits without getting really competitive. Having said that, women can also be very focused and goal-driven."

Caroline is supportive towards potential runners. "Anyone who shows an interest in running I have encouraged. I often download the-couch-to-5km program for them to follow and offer to come running."

She has appreciated the support and encouragement she has received from others. "The best experience involving running is being encouraged by much faster and more talented runners to participate in longer distances such as the half marathon and to train to the best of my abilities. Also, the realisation that slower runners are still real runners is one of my best experiences involving running. On the whole, my experiences with running have been pretty positive. Running is an important part of my life. It makes me feel good."

CHAPTER 35
Great legs are a good enough reason to run

"I haven't worked out what makes it a good run - if I did I'd plan to only have good runs."

Cathy Sheaff, a 39-year-old mother of three, began running about six years ago when a friend convinced her to participate with him and another friend in a triathlon. "He said that he wanted to do the Noosa Tri in teams and also that we were all getting older and he wanted to try to get healthy," Cathy says.

Cathy did the run leg of the Noosa triathlon in the team, while her two friends did the swim and cycle respectively, and enjoyed the experience so much that she did the same in the Mooloolaba triathlon. An annual tradition was born. In the past two years she has also competed in the Gold Coast half marathon. Her reason to run is simple: it makes her feel good.

When preparing for races she runs five times a week, following one of Pat Carroll's online training diaries for the Gold Coast half marathon and she sticks to her program. "I have this printed on the back of my pantry door. I know when I'm meant to run and for how long so I can plan my week around these. I follow my training diary and make sure I fit all runs in. Friends always praise me for being able to go out and run. I pretty much try not to miss one. I hate running on the first couple of days of my period, so I would miss a run then," Cathy says.

Skipping a session does not make her feel guilty, in line with her no-nonsense approach to running in general. "I sometimes miss it. I always feel fat when I have missed a couple of runs. Running doesn't really mean anything to me, I just like to run. Running helps my legs look great," she says.

Cathy always runs alone, wearing an iPod. She runs regardless of her mood. Training makes her feel better. "When it's a great run I feel pretty good, exhausted but good. A crap run doesn't phase me: it's a crap run, they happen, get over it. I haven't worked out what makes it a good run. If I did I'd plan to only have good runs."

Cathy believes her running affects her quality of life in health and fitness. She also considers herself to be healthy because she runs. "But I've always felt fine and felt I had a good quality of life with or without running."

Becoming a runner has influenced her self-esteem and self-image. "I feel fit and slim when I run regularly and feel good about myself. I will keep running until my body says stop."

A couple of injuries forced her to stop running temporarily. "I pulled a hamstring one year and broke my toe another year. Both times it was very frustrating. I missed the running and feeling fit."

Even though she always runs alone, Cathy has made a few friends through running. She looks to the internet and books in the library for information about the sport. In races Cathy focuses on improving her own times, rather than on beating others. "I am not competitive against anyone else running. It's more about me. I like to try to beat my last time in a race."

Her best experience involving running was completing her first half marathon in a better-than-expected time. "I finished my first half marathon 20 minutes faster than what I thought, or what my family thought I'd do it in."

Her worst experience involving running is unfortunately one that she deals with every run. "After having three kids the old pelvic floors aren't quite what they should be. Having to wear a pad or panty liner every run really, really frustrates me," Cathy says.

CHAPTER 36
A long-time walker picks up her pace
"Running is to me proof that I have willpower - inner strength."

Chris Jones began running in her early 40s, about seven years ago. She was inspired by her brother and his annual participation in Sydney's City to Surf 14-kilometre road race. "I started running after years of just walking for fitness, mostly to improve my fitness. I was overweight back then also. My brother is a very good runner and has always competed in the City to Surf. I jokingly suggested to my fellow walkers - four of us - that we should enter the race. We all started to run in preparation for our first City to Surf. That first one was wonderful: a bunch of women doing the road trip to Sydney to shuffle along with 60,000 other people, hilarious moments. It's a lovely memory. I have only missed one race since," Chris says.

Chris prefers running over any other sport because of its flexibility. "I can do it anywhere - no equipment necessary except really good shoes and a running bra. And it's free. It is also outside."

She does four to five training sessions per week and runs before work. "I am consistent. It fits my schedule well as it's early in the morning. I can't imagine starting my work day without it."

She has many other reasons to appreciate her commitment to the endurance sport. "Running is to me proof that I have willpower - inner strength. It's not easy getting up at 5:40am in the dead of winter in Albury and running with very little clothing on. It also has a social component. I train with a couple of other women. Both are strong, interesting women with great careers so we talk things through, as women do so well. I like being this fit and enjoy discussing my running with other runners. I love the way running is the same to the elite athlete as it is to shufflers like me. We experience the same issues."

Chris has made new friends through running, though has also lost touch with the friends she used to walk with. "Running is a great way of connecting with like-minded people. I possibly have lost friends because of running. The ones I walked with originally I rarely see these days."

Generally she finds family and friends encouraging. "Most people are supportive of my running. I am single, though I have two adult sons who are very proud of my fitness. They do laugh at me at times. They think I am mad in winter and early Sunday morning runs just leave them speechless. So I guess they don't fully understand what it means to me, only other runners seem to get it."

Becoming a runner has made a big difference to her life. "I know I have changed since I started running. I have grown in confidence. I am very proud of my fitness. I believe the boys would agree with this. It has impacted on my life in other areas too. Being a runner is a lifestyle for sure."

Chris has days when her training or races feel great. "I feel exhilarated after completing a good run, so pleased with myself and so high. Life looks, seems and feels better. If I had a great run my mood is boosted for the day. A great run has meant I moved at a good pace, that I ran solidly for the allotted time which is 45 minutes usually, that I did the hills well and finished with some energy still left in the tank. It is more mental than physical for sure."

Like any runner, she also has days when her body doesn't cooperate the way she'd like it to. "When it's a crap run my confidence is decreased. I am annoyed with myself. Crap runs are a sign of a lack of preparation, late night, lousy food, alcohol, so I blame myself. If I am not happy with my run I train not harder, but certainly better. My preparation improves."

When she skips training sessions because of overseas holidays for example, she finds returning to training difficult at first. "But I am eager to regain the fitness as soon as possible," Chris says.

A bad mood is never a reason for her to skip a run. In fact she is more likely to go because it will improve her frame of mind. She regards running extremely important to her health. "My quality of life is enhanced by running. I work long hours. I manage a retail business plus teach one day a week at TAFE, plus study part-time at uni. Without my fitness I could not cope with my workload. It helps to give direction and discipline."

Chris doesn't follow a training program. "I just get out and do it, though I have considered coaching." She runs with others, as well as alone. "I enjoy my solo runs equally, possibly more at times. When running with others I try to keep up or push past them. One of my training partners – I run two or three days a week with her - is a very strong runner so she pushes me. Though she struggles on hills and I enjoy the hills the most."

Chris enters races including half marathons and is a competitive person, she says. "I am competitive in most aspects of my life such as career."

CHAPTER 37
Too much champagne led to running a marathon
"Running is supreme as it is freedom for body, mind and soul."

Colette Woodliffe, now 38, ran competitively as a kid and teenager. Then she lost touch with the sport before returning to it with a vengeance four years ago. "I have always been interested in sport both as a participant and a spectator. I ran during all my school years representing the school at sprint and longer distances and also the district at cross country. Then I went to university and found beer, cigarettes and guys. Participating was no longer a priority though being part of the crowd watching certainly was."

She resumed running in her mid 30s to get over a relationship. "I broke up with a guy and found that running was fantastic for headspace and a great tonic all-round. A friend also moved over from the UK and one night over too many champagnes suggested I have a crack at a marathon. I love a challenge so I found myself agreeing. And once verbalised there is no going back."

She has stuck with it since then. "Now I run because it's great fitness and I love to be totally free. There is no one to rely on except oneself and the discipline required is character-building. I also decided to join a running club to hang out with equal-minded people. While I do enjoy running on my own I also like a chat. From this, other goals that I never dreamt I could achieve have been set and completed."

Colette also does other sports such as netball, swimming, touch footy, triathlons, boot camp and rowing. "I will pretty much give anything a go. I enjoy them all for their various reasons; netball as I enjoy the team work and passion on court; swimming as it is something I never thought I would be able to do; triathlons as they are a massive challenge; boot camp for the variety. But running is supreme as it is freedom for body, mind and soul."

Usually she runs three to four times a week which includes one long run of at least 15km. "It depends on what else is going on in my mad life at the time or if I am focused on an event. I just completed the [45km] Six Foot Track event so I have cut back and am enjoying wine and being lazy for a while."

She makes running fit into her life, adding that proves difficult at times. "Being an ex-party girl, sometimes it is hard to say no to a social if it is going to affect my running. By no means does running rule my life but it certainly plays a vital role and keeps the body and mind healthy. As I am fairly disciplined by nature I am slowly learning to say no."

The people close to her are supportive of Colette's passion for running and play a "huge" role in keeping her motivated. As for understanding what running means to her, she believes some do. She hasn't changed since she began running, other than looking fitter and having more friends, she says. "I still socialise and enjoy. I don't need to win any races. I just need to be successful by finishing."

Becoming a runner changed her life, Colette says. "It engrained the discipline needed to succeed as I hate failing."

She loves to race. "I am competitive with myself over shorter distances. Over longer distances I like to just survive and enjoy. I am competitive by nature so naturally I want to overachieve."

On days when racing or training seems effortless, she feels like she could run forever and that no one will catch her. "I feel really exhilarated and a constant reminder of how lucky I am."

On days when running is a struggle, she feels annoyed and frustrated with herself. Whether she feels it was a great run or a bad one is more determined by physical factors than mental ones, she says. "I get annoyed when I get aches and pains. It's not fair when I feel great in myself but my body starts complaining. I try not to listen."

A bad session can increase Colette's motivation. "If it is crap due to an injury then I will sulk until I am allowed to run pain-free again. I will continue to cross-train instead and being told I can't do something just motivates me more to do it."

She'll run regardless of her mood. A great run always lifts her spirits and she feels better after a run than she did before. "I can be carried on the euphoria of a great run for weeks. I am still flying high on the Sydney marathon [done six months earlier] and even higher from Six Foot Track. I love telling people about it and encouraging them to consider running. The feeling cannot be shared among all people but fellow runners get it."

She recommends others to start running. "When they tell me I look fit I thank them and say that it's hard work as it certainly isn't genetic. There's no point complaining about one's weight, health, etc."

Colette typically runs alone. "It's the only time I am totally on my own with my own thoughts. However, on longer, more challenging runs I like to run with a gang who can lift you when you are tired and who I can support when they need it too. I like to be led by someone who pushes me. I will not be taking it easy. I will be there to work out but most of all to enjoy. I prefer a mixed group. The social aspect of running definitely plays a role and more so now I am taking part in bigger events."

When she skips a few runs she misses the training. "But I am the queen of planning so as long as time out of running is my choice or I have had time to get my head around the fact that I cannot run for a couple of weeks then it's OK. It's when it is sprung on me that I get frustrated. I always have a deadline of when I am going to pick it back up and tend to have a goal so I am fine to get back in the groove."

Running is very important to her health and the health benefits are among her main motivators to keep it up, she says. Colette considers herself to be healthy because she runs. It is also very important to her self-esteem and self-image. The sport has brought her many great memories and experiences. "There are too many to mention, though finishing the marathon in Sydney and the Six Foot Track to the sounds of my amazing friends cheering me on is something that makes me tingle. And I love a crowd."

Unfortunately she has also suffered running injuries. "I am just dealing with an ITB injury. My biggest fear was being told not to run: I wasn't, so I am happy with that but it has also made me more aware of the mechanics of the human body. I am determined to do my best to do the right thing so I can run for many, many more years."

CHAPTER 38
Once you find the confidence you will surprise yourself

"I ran 18km and I just could not believe it. I knew then that I could do a half marathon and it felt great to realise I had reached a new level."

Deborah Kemp started running in 2006 at the age of 34. She did about 6 kilometres once a week. She stuck to his routine for months before she felt comfortable enough to venture beyond that distance. "It took ages to build up my confidence to try 8 kilometres," Deborah says. The following year she began running more often and increased her distance and could run 24 kilometres comfortably 12 months later.

Deborah started running in an attempt to get fit. "Really I didn't even know if I could do it. I felt that 35 would be a turning point age-wise. In addition, I have occasionally had mild depression and half an hour of exercise three times a week is great physical treatment. So I had a chance to get fit and feel great. When I started to get more serious in 2007 I lost 8 kilograms which was a nice side-effect."

She has gained enough fitness and confidence in her running ability to enter races. "Now I am enjoying the idea of competing. My running goals this year are to do the two Sydney half marathons in less than two hours. This will still be a stretch but is achievable and a good preparation for moving onto a marathon next year."

Deborah loves the efficiency of running and enjoys the camaraderie in the group she trains with. She usually runs three times a week and is considering increasing that frequency. "Running is a great social activity, outdoors and generally easy to do. I train on Tuesday and Thursday evenings and do a long run on Saturday morning. My favourite are bush runs with breakfast at the end."

Deborah is encouraged by her family and friends. She also believes they understand running is important to her. "My current partner is incredibly fit so he is very supportive. My family think I am nuts but envy me all the same.

"On Saturday I met my Mum after a 23km run in the bush and I was a bit muddy having slipped over a couple of times. Mum couldn't believe that I had kept going after falling over. I am not sure how she thought I would otherwise get out of the bush without a phone, money or car. Nevertheless I think she is proud and amazed that her daughter can do such a thing," Deborah says.

Her loved ones believe she has changed since becoming a runner, saying she is more determined, fitter and looks great.

Deborah says that a good run makes her feel light, strong and healthy. "I always find the first 3km the hardest. After that, I must get endorphins released every 10km or so because I just kick along. I always try to finish strong."

She has sessions during which she struggles. "There is no way to explain it but occasionally you can go for a run and your legs are just heavy. The good news is that it is just one run and you know the next one won't be like that. I just accept that it was a tough day and that there is nothing I can do about it. I stick to my usual routine unless I think I am getting sick - then I give myself some time off."

The best sessions are the ones where she feels she has reached a new level in her running. "In a great run you will always give a lot at the end and feel like you have broken a new barrier or hit a new milestone. For example, the first time I ran further than 12km I ran 18km and I just could not believe it. I knew then that I could do a half marathon and it felt great to realise I had reached a new level."

After such a great run she feels proud of her achievement for at least a day and tells everyone she meets about it. She is more likely to train in a good mood and always feels better after a run than she did before. She occasionally skips sessions. "If I skip it is due to other social things or really bad weather. Generally I try not to skip. If I do, I miss it and know I need to get back to the routine soon. It generally surprises me how quickly you can get back to where you left off."

She believes that being fit is a lifestyle choice and running has affected her quality of life. "Health-wise it is great mentally and physically. The health benefits are probably the main reason I do it, followed by the social aspect. I can run on my own but I just don't enjoy it very much. I have a few running buddies, each of whom is a little better than me and I try to keep up. That is the most fun."

Mentally she finds it important to stay near the front of the group she is running with. "I am also a horse rider and I think of myself in horsy terms: I am a lead horse - very happy at the front. I run faster and have my head up. I know if I fall to the back I will find the run harder just by being at the back. I always try to be near the front for this reason."

She is a competitive person by nature which carries over into her running, she says, "but not enough to make me do lots of training on my own." Deborah follows a training program if she is preparing for an event. "Otherwise I am lazy and just go along to the club runs. Being in a club takes some of the thought out of it."

She credits her club, Northside Running Group, with helping her to become a regular runner through a beginners program. "I tell anyone who says they can't run that it is just something to learn and tell them how I did it. Easy." She always looks to her club for any information on running. "Our club NRG has coaches and heaps of experienced runners. They have everything I would need at my level."

Being a runner is important to her self-esteem, she says. The key thing about running for Deborah is that it makes her feel great. "I have been running for just 18 months - a last-ditch attempt to get fit before I get too old. It has been a fantastic experience and I have learned from my fellow runners at NRG that everybody has at least 20 good years of running so it is all on the up and up for me for a few years yet. My running goals this year are two half marathons and perhaps Mt Wilson to Bilpin [a 35km bush run], then all going well a marathon next year. I have the body of a fit 25-year old. My partner bought me size-8 Roxy shorts for the beach."

Deborah may initially have struggled to work up the courage to increase her 6km runs but things have changed. "I am looking forward to an easy City to Surf for the first time ever. Fourteen kilometres is just not a big deal any more."

CHAPTER 39
Running helped me to take on more challenges

"I had a Birmingham hip replacement and went through a stage of maybe never running again which was totally devastating."

Eileen Varty tried running because she sought an exercise regime that would help her to shed weight. "Like a lot of us I was always involved in fitness and the gym but I never seemed to drop any weight," Eileen says. Running did provide the result she was after, allowing her to lose 10 kilograms over the last five years. While she is very happy about her weight loss, she has since found more important motivators that have inspired her to stick with running even after a hip replacement. "I run now as it helps me with my physical and mental wellbeing. Becoming a runner has changed my life in that I take on more challenges in my career and home life as well. I have been running a successful finance business and have two homes as well as being a single mother to two boys over the last six years and I feel running has also helped me achieve these things," she says.

Eileen runs five days per week. She used to keep track of her sessions in log books but not so much since she had hip surgery last year. She simply reserves time for her running because she loves it. "Running means a lot to me. I prefer running over other exercise. I love the challenge and that reward you get after each run with that runner's high. It's not quite the same for me with anything else. It has become just part of my life. Of course there are some days that I may feel a bit sore or down in the dumps but I usually don't have trouble fitting it in somewhere."

Her family is supportive of her training, as much for Eileen's sake as for their own. "They now know that I become a bit difficult to be around if I don't or can't run. I don't think they quite understand what running means to me. My partner ran with me for a while a few years ago but he did not experience the same joys I did.

"He saw it as more of a chore and strangely never experienced the euphoria after a great run. When it's a great run I am euphoric and on a high all day."

Becoming a runner has made Eileen more conscious of her health. "I cut out alcohol completely and focus my diet on helping my fitness. Running has improved the quality of life immensely. Running is extremely important to my health and I always think about the benefits. I do consider myself healthy - running being some of this," she says.

It has also boosted her self-confidence. "Running is very important to my self-esteem and self-image. I don't want to put that weight back on."

Eileen's appreciation of her ability to run has increased since she had to undergo a Birmingham hip replacement surgery eight months ago. For a while she wasn't sure if she would ever be able to run again. Eileen had been training for the 2006 Brisbane marathon. She started the race but severe pain to her hip prompted her to pull out after 32km. "My major injury was osteoarthritis to the hip joint. I had been told that wasn't caused by running though. I went through a stage of maybe never running again which was totally devastating. I started running not long after surgery. Eight months later I am running 35km to 40km per week regularly and I now appreciate that I can run. It has caused me to love running more and to enjoy because I can and not take it so seriously. When it's a crap run I don't beat myself up about it too much. I used to. If I am not happy with my run it doesn't worry me too much. It just motivates me to train a little differently."

If Eileen skips a few sessions she cannot wait to resume her training. "If I miss a few runs because of sickness or travel I am totally grumpy. It doesn't usually take me much to get back into it. I run in any type of mood. I always feel better after a run."

She typically runs alone, especially since her hip surgery. "I prefer to run on my own most of the time as I can get a chance to think about the upcoming day and problems, life. I sometimes run with a friend and it is nice to have a chinwag. The social aspect of running is not that important. I would do it regardless."

Even so, Eileen had made new friends through her running. "The non-running friends I had have become distant as they don't understand why I run. I have always recommended running to friends. Most people think I am nuts and I get the old 'too skinny' comments as well. My best memories involving running are the regular long runs a girlfriend and a mate used to do every Saturday morning. We would try to solve the world's problems and have a laugh along the way. We don't do so much any more as the max distance I can manage with the hip is around 10km at the moment. We would run up to 26km some weeks - it was great."

Eileen is currently not on a training program. "I am not competitive as am I limited now. I may enter a race this year but will not be so stressed about time. The single-most important thing to me is purely being able to run."

CHAPTER 40
Running a marathon was never a consideration
"Many people are amazed when you say have run a marathon."

Elizabeth Adams began running four years ago. She and a few friends had just prepared for and finished walking the 100-kilometre Oxfam Trailwalker. "We were quite fit and wanted to stay that way," Elizabeth says.

Maintaining her fitness is still one of her prime motivators for running but she has discovered other crucial ones along the way. Running has helped improve her quality of life and is very important to her self-image and self–esteem. "Being fit has many spill-over effects. Many people are amazed when you say have run a marathon," she says.

Running is important to her health and she is conscious of its health benefits. She considers herself healthy because she runs. "Very much so - I rarely have a sick day. My heart rate is lower and I feel confident that my weight is good. I have also increased my strength. I am near menopause and am conscious of staying fit and keeping my weight in check," says Elizabeth, who is 49.

She runs twice a week, consistently on Thursday nights and Saturday morning. She also aims to support her running fitness by Pilates classes, swimming and walking to work. Elizabeth doesn't keep track of her runs in a log book but is aware of the distance she covers when she is training for major events with her club, the Northside Running Group. "We have club training logs for the major events like [the 45km] Six Foot Track so I am generally aware of the kilometres."

Her training fits very well into her life, she says. People close to her are supportive of her passion for running. Her 64-year-old husband also runs as do some of her friends. Most friends understand what running means to her, though not all. "It is so foreign to them," Elizabeth says.

Running makes up a significant part of Elizabeth's leisure time and consequently social life, she says. She typically trains with others from her running club and has made new friends through running. "In fact, we spend more time with our new running friends than our old friends. I enjoy running with a mixed group. The social aspect of running is very important. I have made some good friends. We go out socially. I travel interstate and overseas for running events."

When it is a great run Elizabeth feels fantastic. "All is well with the world. You also acknowledge and appreciate the simple things."

If she struggles during a run she just finishes it and doesn't over-think it. "I get over it and make it to the end. Avoid giving up unless you are injured. I simply put it down to a bad day and move on," Elizabeth says.

Mental factors, more so than physical ones, determine whether she feels she's had a great run or a bad one. Occasionally she skips training, usually when she feels her body needs a break. "Sometimes I have a twinge and decide to swim instead. I had three stress fractures in about two years when I started to run. Hopefully I have now conditioned my bones. I haven't suffered an injury for nearly two years."

While she does miss running when she skips sessions, she also knows that a rest now and then doesn't hurt her fitness. Her mood doesn't affect her decision to run. She generally feels better after a run than she did before. "Perhaps I see running as a good opportunity to blow out the cob webs or rid daily frustrations."

She rewards herself for consistent training and reaching goals with a glass of wine or two, she says. Elizabeth enters races, with her favourites being half and full marathons. She says she is not a competitive person.

Elizabeth has recommended others to start running. "I have used my own case as an example of how you can take up running in your mid to late 40s. Running has changed my life significantly. I never saw myself as being a runner. Doing a marathon was never a consideration - until two years ago."

CHAPTER 41
My brother said I wouldn't last training in an ice storm

"I am 48 and in very good shape. My mom says I have the body of a 25-year old. I say, 'Mom, I work really hard at it'."

Jan Roberts began running on January 26, 2000, after she moved from the UK to Australia. "I started running because I had turned 40 the year before in November. In the UK, I had joined the gym and was working out. When I came to Brisbane, there wasn't a gym around the area where we moved and the shore front was absolutely stunning. This inspired me to get out and just run," she says.

Five marathons later, Jan loves her running. "I still do it for the fitness. But I have since moved again and joined a gym so I can cross-train as I have suffered a few injuries last year just by running so much. I hope to never give it up as I am very addicted to it. I love the open air, the time alone and the way I get a high afterwards that I don't get from the gym."

Becoming a runner has lifted Jan's quality of life. "It has made me healthier, mentally and physically. I always think about the health benefits of running. It has also given me a lot of confidence, especially after running marathons as I think I could do anything I set my mind to do," Jan says.

To Jan running means freedom. "It is something that no one can take away from me, except for injuries, and the freedom as I run - that whole feeling of being in my head and forgetting that I am actually running. I truly prefer running over any other sport or exercise. It is something I can do anywhere at anytime, by myself, all I need are my runners, and it is all mine."

She typically runs four to five times a week consistently. Last year injuries curtailed her run training. "I went to the gym to make up for any loss of fitness. This year I am back to running four to five times per week or more. I have at least one day rest from everything," Jan says.

She usually trains early in the day. "I make running one of my main priorities. You just have to do that, otherwise it would fall by the wayside. So I run in the mornings when I get up."

People close to Jan are very supportive of her running. But that wasn't always the case. "My husband is very supportive. He is a sporty person, so he understands. Although he doesn't run, he plays other sports. My first husband hated it for some reason. He just didn't seem to understand that the running was my time. I think he was jealous."

Jan says her husband is probably the only person close to her who completely understands what running means to her. "My daughter wouldn't as she is only 11. My husband does, but my mother wouldn't understand really. I think I have made them realise how important exercise is. I am 48 and in very good shape. My mom says I have the body of a 25-year old. I say, 'Mom, I work really hard at it'."

On the days Jan has a great run she feels powerful. "I feel like I could conquer the world. I feel brilliant for a few hours afterwards." On those days that running feels hard she just accepts that it does. "I think, 'Maybe I will conquer the world another day'. No actually I just think, 'Bugger, bad run, oh well'."

For Jan a bad run is usually determined by physical aspects such as feeling tired, pain or sluggish, rather than mental ones. She never dwells on those days. "I never think about skipping a session just because I had a bad run the day before. I know each run is different and that is what motivates me to get out there and do it."

When Jan skips a few runs she misses it. "One day is OK but two or more and I start getting cranky. I find it easy to get back into it." She'll run regardless of her mood and typically feels better after a run. "If I am in a bad mood I will just say to myself, 'Run what you feel like running'. And I usually end up having a good run."

At times she has kept track of her training in a log book. "But I found that I stopped as I got injured and haven't returned to logging my runs. Plus my personality isn't a list-person. It is interesting though to look back and think, 'Man I ran that much in that short a time'."

Jan trains by herself. She hasn't made new friends because of running and hasn't lost any either. She hasn't recommended others to start running. The social aspect of running is not important to her, although she enjoys being with other runners at marathons. "I love running alone. I have run with other people probably a total of four times in my whole running career."

She doesn't follow a program. "I feel that would ruin the fun of running for me. I do sort of, if I am going to be running a marathon but not full-on and strict."

Jan is selective in the races she enters – she only does marathons. "I don't like the short races. I suppose I don't really like running fast. I feel competitive in a race, definitely. I don't like it when people pass me. Also in my career I am competitive but mostly with myself."

USA-born Jan is pretty determined which does not always work to her advantage such as three years ago when she visited her family in her hometown in Indiana in winter. "There was an ice storm and I wanted to go out for a run because we had a long journey ahead of us back to Australia. My brother said I wouldn't last out there 20 minutes. Of course I had to last longer to show him. I lasted about 45 minutes and absolutely froze. I thought I was going to die of hypothermia or something. Honestly. It took me forever to get warm."

Her best experience involving running was her most recent marathon. "I had such a good race and felt wonderful afterwards. I was on a high for days and couldn't sleep the night after I ran - I was so thrilled."

Being a runner is a lifestyle for Jan. "It is something I can do that a lot of people can't or won't. I really have no age in mind of when I will stop."

CHAPTER 42
Running brings freedom and confidence to my spirit

"I not only think about the health benefits, I also feel them as my body changes and I become stronger."

Laura How, 27, started running about 15 months ago because she wanted to lose weight. She followed a training program designed by a coach. To support her drive she put $1 for every kilometre she ran into a money box. The distance she covered increased steadily as Laura trained for and completed the Gold Coast marathon within seven months of taking up the sport. "As I became a better runner I found the $1-per-kilometre scheme hard to afford. When I eventually broke open the money box I had hundreds and hundreds of dollars," she says.

Laura used the funds to help pay for her Gold Coast marathon trip – she booked five-star accommodation and a massage. These days she rewards herself for special accomplishments in training and racing with chocolate and ice cream.

Weight control is still an important motivator for her running but she also has found others. "I do still run today to maintain my weight but also because I enjoy running as a pastime and feel great about myself after doing a long and strong run. Running has enhanced my life by giving me a healthy hobby that I really enjoy. I not only think about the health benefits, I also feel them as my body changes and I become stronger. It is a means to stay healthy and a great stress reliever when I am having a bad day. It fills me with a great sense of achievement after completing a good run or a long race," Laura says.

Her active lifestyle is important to Laura and has prompted changes to accommodate her training. "It's more like how does my life fit around my running? I get tired quite a lot especially in summer and it means that I choose not to go out and party with friends as much as I used to. Most of my runs are done between 5am and 7am or 4:30pm and 7pm as I work fulltime. This can sometimes upset my partner especially when he has to cook his own dinner as I am not home, or when I am home I couldn't be bothered cooking."

Laura's weekly training routine includes four runs. She also swims and cycles but says running is her preferred way to exercise. Laura follows a training program, especially if she is preparing for a race. While she generally aims to do all her sessions, this doesn't always happen. She says there are many reasons or excuses including the weather being too hot, cold or wet, as well as tiredness and lack of time because of special occasions or work. She feels very guilty for skipping training and misses it. "It is hard to get back into it but very rewarding when I do."

While training for her first marathon she logged the distance she ran each session in a diary as well as how she felt afterwards. "This was mostly for my running coach as I was training for a marathon and he wanted to see how I was going. I found it a lot of work," Laura says.

The people close to Laura applaud her passion for running, especially her training buddy Kim. "Most people are supportive. Some can not believe the distances I have run and admire it. I have a running partner Kim who is especially supportive, and we run with and for each other. We also have a running coach who is always there to encourage us and keep us motivated."

Even so, not everyone understands what running means to Laura. "Kim does but generally friends and family do not. I feel that running is quite a personal thing and there are a lot of emotions associated with working so hard and pushing yourself - the glory when you do well and the disappointment when you don't."

Having Kim to train and race with is very important to Laura. "Through the different races and experiences we have shared we have become quite close and we often comment that we couldn't have done any of it without each other.

"Initially we used to run side by side. We now set off for runs together but run at our own paces. It is good to know that there is someone else out there with you although we are not necessarily running side by side. If it was not for Kim I would not be as committed to running as I am. We motivate and rely on each other."

Laura finished her first marathon with her best friend by her side which is so far her best experience involving running. "We felt invincible," she says.

And that is generally what accomplishments in training or racing do for Laura. "When it's a great run I smile on the inside - generally because I have no energy left to physically smile. Words can't really express it, I just feel happy."

A great run boosts her mood for a day. The factor that determines where she feels it has been a great or a bad session is generally based on the time and distance she has run, rather than how she felt physically. "If I have really struggled but achieved a PB then it is a good run."

She feels disappointed if she struggles during her training or in a race. "Usually it is because I have been lazy and haven't run in a while or because I am not sufficiently hydrated and fuelled. I only have myself to blame and it gives me renewed determination to improve. I try to make sure that I am not in that situation again and then I try to become more consistent with diet, fluids and sessions."

Laura will run regardless of her mood, especially when her training partner Kim is counting on her and her coach makes her feel bad for thinking about skipping a session. She never regrets going for a run. "There's no question, I always feel better after a run than before," she says.

Laura cherishes the time spent with Kim and the other new friends she has made because of running. Even so, Laura doesn't consider the social aspect of running important. "Running is me-time, time to think and be in my own space."

When Laura trains with others she sticks to her own pace. "I am happy to take it easy. I don't like holding people back so I am often the first to say, `You guys can run off ahead if you like. Don't worry about me'."

Becoming a runner has not been without setbacks for her. "I once had blisters so bad that I couldn't walk for three days and was on antibiotics. This was three weeks before the Gold Coast marathon so I was pretty determined anyway. After training for the marathon and running it, I ended up with a very bad iron deficiency which in turn made it impossible for me to fight off colds and flues. I was sick for five weeks and could not run. Somehow I managed to get back into it, definitely helped by being supported by an eager running partner."

She enters five to six local running races a year. She doesn't consider herself to be competitive as a runner. "I have only been running for 15 months and know that I need to be running for a lot longer to even consider myself a good runner. I am more competitive in team sports, I only ever run against and for myself."

Laura believes women approach running in a different way than men do. "Men are quite competitive about running and women run to improve themselves."

She has recommended running to others. "I do encourage it although I know that physically it is not the best sport for everyone. I just tell them that if I can do it then anyone can."

Laura says she has changed since she began running. "It has made me more driven in all aspects of my life and given me goals, hopes and dreams. I believe that I have more confidence in myself. I feel that I have become quieter too. I go out less and spend a lot more time at home relaxing."

Running plays a role in her self-esteem and self-image as it helps to make her feel and look good. The single-most important thing about running for Laura is "the freedom and confidence it brings to my spirit. I hope to run for as long as I can. I have seen people at events in their 60s and 70s - I hope that that is me one day."

CHAPTER 43
Following a training program helps me focus
"My husband says I'm much nicer after I have been running."

Manda Milling had been running intermittently since 1995. In 2005, the then-43-year-old decided to, as she puts it, crank it up and joined Pat Carroll. Manda ran two half marathons in 2006. Over the years her reasons to run have changed. She got into the sport to lose weight and to improve her health. The social side was also an important driver. "I ran with girlfriends and we would chat and have a great breakfast afterwards. It was very sociable. I had done a lot of aerobics in the 1980s, who didn't, and thought I would give running a go," Manda says.

After the birth of her son in 2002, Manda found that running best suited her new schedule. "It was the most time-efficient and effective form of exercise I could do within a limited window of opportunity."

Nowadays her main driver for running is her desire to stay healthy. "Much more so now that I am 46 and I have a husband, a child and a business. People rely on me. It's not as sociable anymore as it's more difficult to pre-arrange with family commitments."

Being a runner helps slow down the ageing process and provides a general sense of wellbeing, she says. "Running to me means a sense of empowerment as I know I am fitter than a lot of women, or even people, at my age. It gives me a feeling that I can do things I couldn't in my earlier years. It's self-satisfaction. It's a challenge you never quite get on top of. It's also being part of a wider community, even if you don't know the participants."

Manda does her training early in the morning to avoid running out of time later in the day through other commitments. "It's a lot easier for me to fit it in around work and family if I run in the morning. If I don't get out then, my window slams shut."

Manda aims to do four sessions a week which she manages to do consistently if she is focused on a specific goal or race. "I haven't been as consistent during the past year, so it's once to twice per week. I am a goal-oriented runner."

She keeps track of her runs, particularly when she follows a training program developed for her by Pat Carroll. She also cross-trains with a group, led by a trainer, once a week and power-walks.

The people close to her are supportive of her passion for running. "My husband is. He says I'm much nicer after I have been running. My parents think it's too hard on my body. But then, they don't live with me. A lot of my friends do some form of exercise on a regular basis too."

She believes they "mostly" understand what running means to her. Manda says running has benefited her through weight loss and by broadening her horizons. "My hips are smaller. It's another interest other than work and family and that's important."

Running can make her feel amazing. A great session will boost her mood for days or longer. "When it's a great run I feel indescribable. When I completed those two half marathons I really felt such a level of achievement. I didn't know I could even run that far and recover so well."

She believes more mental than physical aspects determine whether she feels it has been a great run or a bad session. "You just aren't in the zone. Physically you don't really feel it until afterwards anyway. When it's a crap run I am very hard on myself and do have a tendency to beat myself up over these things. But then I know the next run can be completely different."

She always feels better after a run than she did before, physically and mentally, and never lets her mood interfere with her training. "Running doesn't depend on my moods. I'm not that moody really. It's more about having to stick to my schedule. I try not to skip training sessions. If I do, it's because I'm tired at the end of the working week. Fridays are the days that get skipped."

If she skips a few days she misses her training. "I do miss it, I feel very sluggish and guilty. I lose some confidence that I can do it again."

While running is important to her self-esteem and self-image, it doesn't define her. "I see it as an important outside interest that has flow-on benefits. Running makes me more alert and I look better in my clothes. It also gives me some bragging rights. It also means I can indulge in my other passion: food."

Manda prefers to run with others, rather than alone. "I would prefer to have a running buddy more often than not. I find running solo all the time a bit lonely. I enjoy mixed groups a lot, but I don't have a preference really, as long as it's someone. The social aspect of running is very important. It's a great bonus."

While she isn't following a training program right now, she generally does: Pat Carroll's. "If I don't have one I tend to lose focus, also I know that I have more chance of avoiding injury when following an expert's program."

She has suffered injuries that stopped her from running, plantar fasciitis mainly. The forced layoff was frustrating and she was keen to get healthy again so she could resume her training.

Manda enters races as they help her to stay focused and motivated in her training. She considers herself competitive. "That can be my undoing. I tend to be a competitive person by nature. I work in a competitive field and industry. When I am in a race I measure myself against other women my age or older - not the elites, I'm not that masochistic. It does spur me on to try harder."

While her most cherished memories involving running are the two half marathons she completed in 2006, her worst is her first attempt at a half marathon a year earlier. "I had the runner's trots - you don't want to know the details - doing my first half marathon in September 2005. I was not able to finish and tried to find a taxi in the middle of the course to get home. All the roads were shut. It still pains me to think of it."

Becoming a runner changed her life. Manda had never been that sporty which make her accomplishments as a runner even more satisfying. "It gives you a sense of achievement. You think, 'Wow, I did that'. The single-most important thing about running for me is feeling healthy and looking good."

She has recommended others to start running. "They always tell me they can't run but find that they can. It's time efficiency and the good it does your hips."

CHAPTER 44
Running made me realise that I like to compete

"I like the feeling of satisfaction that I get when I complete a significant race such as a 10km or a half marathon."

Margo McLay began running in January 2007 at the age of 47 for several reasons: to get over a broken heart, lose weight and because she had agreed to run 10km as a team member in a triathlon. "I panicked and then started practising," Margo says.

She now also competes regularly in running races and has completed one half marathon in less than two hours. "The reason that I have continued running is different. I now find I have running group friends, I like the fact that running is the best fat-burner and I like the feeling of satisfaction that I get when I complete a significant race such as a 10km or a half marathon. Because of running I think that I have grasped that I like to be competitive."

A very important benefit of running are increasingly toned legs, Margo says. "Running means that I can keep my weight at bay. If I keep my running up in a dedicated fashion, it is highly likely that the tone and shape of my legs will improve significantly, and that would make me a very happy woman."

She also cycles and does boot camps. "I actually like the variety rather than 100 percent running but running is the area that I can effectively compete in. I am very self-competitive. I am not so interested in competing with others."

Margo "more or less" follows a training program and believes that is something she could improve upon. When she is focused, which is typically when she is preparing for a race, she runs three times a week. "Mostly, I need a scary goal to keep me regimented."

Doing her training early in the day works best for her. "Because I exercise first thing in the morning it fits in. Running is fairly time-efficient as well."

The people close to her think she is mad but are nonetheless impressed with her training and racing. Margo says they probably don't understand what running means to her – and says that is fine.

Whether she feels that it has been a great or a bad run is determined by the time she took to complete it. "I am either better or worse than my PB. I generally don't feel very good but I feel quite satisfied about an hour later. Even if it is a crap run I think, 'At least I have done it'."

A session in which she improves her time boosts her mood. "I feel brilliant and very clever and terribly proud of myself - and sore."

She is initially hard on herself if she is not happy with her run. "But then I get over it and get back in the joggers. I then book myself into something [a race] as a motivator to start practising again."

If she skips her training she feels guilty. Even so, she regards missing a few runs as something that is part and parcel of a busy lifestyle. "I am a pragmatist and if I can't, I can't. If I have been bad and gained weight, after a holiday for example, I dread Day 1 back in the joggers. After the first day I accept the pain quite readily and start the routine once again."

She feels "much, much better" after a run than she did before but is more likely to run when she is in a good mood than when she is in a bad one. She says that running improves her quality of life significantly and is very important to her health. "I think about the health benefits a lot. They motivate me. My health is better if I run rather than if I am not running."

Her self-esteem and self-image have improved. "Running affects my body shape significantly, for the better, and hence my self-esteem and self-image are enhanced."

She likes training with others and has made new friends because of the sport. "I like mixed groups better. Men are less noisy than women."

Margo has recommended others to start running and often makes them commit to doing a specific race as motivation. "I get them to book into an event, and then organise the dinner and drinks around the event. That generally gets their interest."

CHAPTER 45
The healthier my body the better my life

"People think it is too hard but until you start you don't realise that it isn't that difficult at all and you don't have to be fast to be a runner."

Rhonda LeBrocque began running in January 2002 at the age of 40 shortly after she moved to a new town. She had been playing netball, basketball and touch before her relocation. "I met a group of running women that met every Tuesday and Thursday morning for a run and swim so I decided to give it a go. When I began running I had a few extra kilograms to shift and I found that I was able to lose weight and get fit, more so than when I was doing all my team sports. And even though I had never been a runner I realised that I actually enjoyed it," Rhonda says.

She has been running since and completed the Gold Coast half marathon twice. "I enjoy running a lot more than any other activity that I do. I occasionally swim, cycle, go to the gym and do other activities but I always run as it gives the best feeling afterwards. You have a great day if you start it with a run."

Rhonda runs three to four times a week. Her group typically runs about 7km on Tuesdays and Thursdays, about 5km on Saturdays and up to 10km on Sundays. "I am very consistent," she says.

She follows a training program when she is training for a specific race and then sticks to it religiously. If she does skip a session she feels guilty. "And then that seems to set the mood for the day."

She makes sure she gets her run done first thing in the morning, which means 6am on weekdays. On the weekends she will sleep longer before getting up to do her training. The people close to Rhonda are supportive of her passion for running. She believes they understand what running means to her, especially her husband. "My husband runs with my group now and sometimes my children run as well. They are all very supportive. My kids think I am a fanatic."

A good run leaves her elated. "The feeling after a great run is so high you wonder why it can't be like that every time you run."

A session during which she struggles leaves her feeling disappointed. "I try to work out why it was bad and why I run, and whether I need to get fitter or lose weight especially if I have a few bad runs in a row. But then I also feel determined to run better next time."

A disappointing run doesn't hurt her mood as she pats herself on the back for getting out there. "Had I stayed in bed then my mood would be bad. It makes me more determined to keep going as I often relate bad runs with fitness even though I know it isn't that."

Rhonda says there may be more physical than mental aspects that determine whether she feels she has had a bad run or a great one. "With a great run you could just keep going. You feel you can go faster, harder and stronger. Then when you have finished you just think, 'Wow I feel good, you wouldn't think I just ran 7km or whatever distance. My mood is lifted after every run but definitely after a good run. It makes you think this is what I run for."

When she skips a few runs she misses her training. "I enjoy the rest but I am also busting at the bit to hit the pavement again. Sometimes I find it hard for the first few runs back, but I have a very supportive running group so we are constantly encouraging each other." Her mood doesn't influence her decision to train. "If I run when I am in a bad mood it certainly cheers me up."

Rhonda considers herself to be healthy because she runs. "Running is important to your health and I constantly think about the benefits. I am sure I am a lot healthier for the life I lead." She also regards running extremely important for her self-esteem. "I think it makes you feel you can do anything."

Rhonda prefers training with others over solo runs and says the social aspect is essential. "I probably wouldn't run if my group of friends didn't. I don't enjoy running by myself much. I prefer to run with girlfriends. However I often run with my husband. I enjoy running with him but he is faster than I am. It is better to run with someone your own speed."

Running is conducive for a good heart-to-heart with her girlfriends. "During our run we solve the problems of the world, marriage, children or any other things that come up. It is a great counselling session when you are down or things just aren't going your way."

Rhonda has remained injury-free except for a twisted ankle during training for her first half marathon. "I had to rest for a few weeks so I took up water running with a buoyancy device. I was very annoyed and very anxious to get back into it."

Rhonda has completed several 10km races, two half marathons, two City to Surfs in Sydney and many local fun runs. She says she is not competitive. "Until I did my first half marathon I didn't even consider myself a real runner. I am a bit competitive with my children and their sport, but I don't see myself as a fast runner or as a threat to beat many people so I am happy to plod along and finish."

Her best experience involving running was finishing her first half marathon. "And thinking how wonderful I was. It was then that I really considered myself a runner," Rhonda says. .

Becoming a runner has changed her life. "I love running and feel disappointed if I miss a run. I feel healthy and often wonder why not everyone runs. People think it is too hard but until you start you don't realise that it isn't that difficult at all and you don't have to be fast to be a runner."

She has recommended running to others. "I tell many people to start out by running between lamp posts and then two lamp posts and build it up slowly. I try to make it sound achievable and invite them to join our morning running group."

Being a runner is a lifestyle which is important to Rhonda. "The healthier I keep my body the better my life will be and also longer hopefully."

CHAPTER 46
Running means fitness, looking good and staying young

"He encouraged me to try the China Coast half marathon and I thought he was nuts. But I did it."

Ros Holcombe started running in 1995 at the age of 31. Two years earlier she had moved from Sydney where she swam, surfed and walked for fitness to Hong Kong. She had tried running before but hadn't taken to it. The lack of clean swimming water in Hong Kong's pools and ocean prompted her to join a gym and run on the treadmill during her lunch breaks in an effort to stay fit. "My boss was very encouraging and eventually I joined a local running club and started doing 5km races. He encouraged me to try the China Coast half marathon and I thought he was nuts. But I did it, not knowing the course we raced was the toughest half course I've ever seen," Ros says.

Since then she has completed numerous running races including the Great Ocean Road marathon, her favourite so far. Her motivation for running has evolved. "I started running to get fit. Along the way I have discovered the challenge of pushing myself to run longer distances I would never have dreamed of running in the 1990s. After seven marathons I still get an enormous sense of achievement from completing a marathon. So I run for fitness, the challenge, and for vanity because running keeps me looking young and sexy."

Ros, who has since moved back to Sydney, runs three times a week if she is not preparing for a specific race. She runs five times a week and keeps track of her training in a log book when she is focused on competing in an event.

Ros also swims and cycles. She has completed a few triathlons including the Port Macquarie half Ironman. "I love ocean swimming but running is the best fat-burner, you can do it anywhere and compared with cycling it's safe and hassle free and there are always scenic places to run," she says.

Ros has great and not-so-great running sessions. During the former she wants to keep going. "I feel totally energised and in tune with my body." If she struggles in a session, she feels sluggish and can only manage a slow pace. "I don't feel like going on past the distance I have determined at the start. I just accept that you have bad days occasionally and go back the next day to try again."

Both mental and physical aspects determine whether she feels it has been a great run or a bad one. A superb session usually lifts her spirits for the whole day. She never lets her mood affect her decision to train and always feels better after a run than she did before. When she skips a few runs she misses the training. "I start to feel sluggish and more negative. It's easy to get back into it again by starting with an easy goal of 20 minutes, then once you start you keep going."

She doesn't feel guilty for skipping sessions because she typically only does when work gets in her way.

Running is important to her health, she says. She considers herself to be healthy because she runs. By healthy she means the absence of ill health as well as a positive frame of mind and a proper body weight.

Becoming a runner has her made more confident and helped her realise she could achieve things she once thought impossible. It has improved her self-esteem and self-image. "It helps me to look younger than I am and stay slim."

Ros has made new friends because of running. She has recommended others to start running and tries to encourage them by offering to take them for easy sessions and pointing out races and race calendars. Even so, the social aspect of running is not very important to her and she prefers to run alone.

She doesn't consider herself competitive in running or in other aspects of life. She does reward herself for consistent training or reaching certain goals. "I bought a topaz ring for completing the Port Macquarie half Ironman."

Ros has suffered injuries because of running and was determined to get better so she could resume her training. The single-most important thing about running for her is the mental lift it gives her. "Running means fitness, looking good, staying young. A great start to the day as it energises you. I go mad if I don't run."

CHAPTER 47
Running is a priority in my life because I make it one

"Sometimes I will feel exhausted before a run but when I get back I am completely energised."

Shannon Daley had been doing some unstructured running for years. She started training properly in 2001 when she took up triathlon to help out a friend who was studying for a Level-2 Triathlon coaching certificate. "One of her course requirements was to develop a structured training program for someone and follow their development over a six-month period. We were at the pub one night and she mentioned it to me. Before I knew it I was on a training program to start sprint distance triathlons. Although the reason I got into triathlon was to help out my friend, it was no stretch to exercise and be active as I had always done some form of activity and fitness. It just varied and wasn't especially running," Shannon says.

These days she is focused on running and trains six days a week consistently: she runs on four to five days and cycles on an indoor trainer on two days. "I am concerned about getting injured otherwise I would be running seven days per week. The body just isn't up for it."

Shannon prefers running over swimming and cycling. "Running is quick, cheap and gets the best results for minimum time spent doing it."

Shannon used to log her training in a diary but hasn't done so in the past 12 months. "I am trying to just enjoy my training and not be so focused on the miles so I have not been keeping a log book recently."

Running is a priority in her life. "I will always make sure I have time to train even if I am away with work or on holidays. I train early in the morning so it doesn't infringe on me doing other things. It possibly means I don't have as many late nights as I am always thinking about how it will impact my run the next day – sad, I know."

"To me running means I get to eat whatever I like, I feel fit and healthy, I get to socialise through my training with friends and I remain focused on goals."

A great training session or race leaves Shannon feeling energised, motivated, determined, excited and hungry and will lift her spirits for hours. "For the whole day I feel great. I feel like I have deserved whatever it is I do, for example great food, resting, partying, whatever. Each day is a new day however and it's a fresh start the next morning and requires another run."

A session in which she struggles makes her feel human. "It's very difficult to maintain peak energy levels day in day out. If I have a crap run then I feel like my next run will have to be a great one to make up for it."

Shannon believes physical factors rather than mental ones determine how she feels about her run. "Your body just gets tired. It's hard not to let a physically-hard run drag your mental run down too. Luckily from experience now I know not to think one bad run means it's all over. Energy levels vary so greatly from day to day."

While Shannon is very consistent with her training, she also keeps a close eye out for signs that she might need to take a break. "I stick to my routine no matter what. I know lots of people who train more if they have a bad run or race. I'm the opposite: I think it could be a sign to train less and give your body a rest."

She simply makes time for her run training. "I never miss a run due to travel. There's always a road to run on and always enough hours in the day if you want. If I'm sick then I definitely take time off and can't wait to get back into my training when I'm better. Sometimes after being sick though it takes a few runs to feel 100 percent on track again," Shannon says.

Consequently she doesn't let her mood interfere with her training, though she's more likely to run harder if she is in a bad mood. A run always makes her feel better. "Sometimes I will feel exhausted before a run but when I get back I am completely energised."

Running underpins her lifestyle. "I have a great quality of life through being healthy and also the friends you meet through training. Others may disagree and say I'm boring and miss out on partying."

Shannon says she definitely takes the health benefits of running into consideration. "I work in the health industry and know all about the complications obesity, smoking, and lack of exercise can cause. I'm healthy because I run but also because I'm a healthy weight, I eat well and I don't drink excessive alcohol."

CHAPTER 48
Running at my pace sustains my love for the sport

"I love how I feel as a result of running - mentally and physically. It's a real outlet for me. It helps me keep a positive perspective on life."

Sharon Varley took up running in 1992 at the age of 38. "I was dating someone who ran every day and thought I'd give it a try in the hopes that we could do it together. I also really liked the small group of friends she ran with," she says.

Sharon now trains two to three times a week consistently, and considers running a top priority in her life. Her motivation to run has changed. "I love how I feel as a result of running - mentally and physically. It's a real outlet for me. It helps me keep a positive perspective on life."

She also participates in other sports and likes to have a balance of those. Running does provide a clear benefit. "Running is the easiest in terms of scheduling. Running means keeping fit, a social circle of friends, time out of doors and time to myself for reflection."

The people close to Sharon are supportive of her passion for running and try to understand what it means to her, she says.

She has good days and bad days when it comes to her training. A solid session boosts her mood for at least a day. "When it's a great run I feel happy, like I can do anything, lucky, grateful that I'm healthy and can still run at my age. When it's a crap run I feel disappointed and tired," she says.

For Sharon the difference between feeling that it has been a great run or a bad one lies in whether she struggled physically the whole time. "During a bad run, for example, I have legs like lead, it's hard to breathe, my knees ache or I couldn't keep up with the group. It doesn't ruin my day. I just try to figure out what I could have done to make it better, such as more sleep, supplements, more stretching or icing my knees after a run," Sharon says.

She is more likely to run in a good mood, although sometimes she will run to get rid of a down-mood. She always feels better after a run. When she skips a few runs she misses it and is concerned about getting back into it. "There's a bit of anxiety about the first run back. Will it be hard? Will I struggle?"

Her health is a significant consideration. "Running is extremely important to my health and I do think about the health benefits all the time. Running contributes to my overall health and fitness."

She enjoys running alone as well as with others. "I do a mix. I run at least once a week by myself and at least once with group."

When Sharon runs with a group she is usually happy to hang back and take it easy. She likes to talk with other runners if the type of training session allows it.

"I am likely to chat when I've got the breath to do so. Serious chats happen - it depends on whether I or someone else has the need on the day."

Sharon enters running races and prefers long, off-road runs. She doesn't consider herself a competitive person. "I'm not a natural runner and it doesn't come easy. I'm just happy that I can run fairly well. If I go at a pace that suits me, then I don't get frustrated and keep my love for it alive."

CHAPTER 49
Running adds energy to my life and brightens my moods
"It taught me that hard work and patience pay off and I apply it to all aspects of my life."

Stephanie Yeung began running in 1998 at the age of 24 because she was preparing for a triathlon with her work colleagues. Over the years, she slowly but surely progressed from completing her first sprint triathlon to qualifying for and competing at the annual Ironman World Championships in Kona, Hawaii, in 2005. Initially her running was simply a part of her triathlon training. Now retired from competing in those to refocus on her successful and time-consuming career, her running is motivated by other factors. "Running adds energy to my life and brightens my moods. I still run as part of my mental health program to keep fit and as a distraction from work," she says.

Stephanie still cycles for fitness but prefers running for its simplicity. "It is the easiest and most convenient thing to do. All I need are my running shoes."

Stephanie is usually consistent with her training. She runs two to three times a week, typically aiming for up to 10km each time. She only follows a training program and increases the distance when she has a goal in mind. The people close to her are very supportive of her passion for running, with the exception of her mother. "Mum worries that doing too much exercise will hurt the body," she says.

Stephanie loves the feeling of a great run. "The body feels strong and I have a treat afterwards to reward myself. I don't usually have crap runs, as being able to run now is an added bonus."

A solid run will boost her mood for at least for a few hours. If her session doesn't go well Stephanie will try to find the reason for it.

"It will make me think why did I have a bad run, for example, do I have my period; did I have a big night; am I injured; am I just really tired? And I try to understand what and how they affect my running."

Stephanie occasionally skips training sessions because of illness or work. She only feels guilty when she misses a lot of training. "I always ease myself back to a slow and short run first."

She feels better after a run. She's more likely to run when she's in a good mood. She considers herself to be healthy because she runs. Running adds to her self-esteem. "It helps a bit because it does control the weight, but not to an extent of beauty-conscious," Stephanie says.

She enjoys running alone as well as with others. "The social aspect of running is not that important but it's nice to mix with people who have a similar interest."

She has recommended others to start running and tells them about the health benefits. Her best experience involving running is training in amazing scenery. Twisting her ankle during a run in the dark is her worst experience involving running.

Stephanie says she has a competitive streak. "Definitely when I was running and training for Ironman. Overall, I consider myself quite competitive but only within myself," she says.

She expects to keep running as long as she is able to. Becoming a runner changed her life. "It taught me that hard work and patience pay off at the end and I apply it to all aspects of my life."

CHAPTER 50
Feeling fabulous helps get us out the door now
"Being only a novice, I found any sort of training sessions a form of hell and motivating myself to get out the door really tough."

Sue Cameron started running with her husband after they suddenly realised their once-active lifestyle had become a very sedentary one. "After the highlights of getting married and the honeymoon we found ourselves on the couch eating and getting fatter and fatter. What was going on? We were really active people. Was it just winter or the downhill slide into married life and health oblivion?"

They decided it was time to do something about it and get fit. "We started running together. My husband could run and I never had. My first run of 17 minutes to the local footy oval, around it and home nearly killed me. Being only a novice, I found any sort of training sessions a form of hell and motivating myself to get out the door and into the weather - whatever that would be - really tough."

While Sue and her husband have struggled at times with making their training a consistent part of their lives, the way they feel after finishing training sessions and races draws them back into their training routine. "Every time we went and pushed ourselves we felt fabulous. We would get into a great routine and then something would throw it out and back to the couch. Hang on, what are we doing? Where are my runners? After much discussion we have come to the conclusion that it is all about the high - the 7 minutes of euphoria after finishing a race or a hard session."

At the time of writing Sue was 30 weeks pregnant with her third child. "I look longingly at the runners go by. I can't wait to start again, I am so jealous. I am still a novice but I want the 7 minutes, I want to feel strong and alive rather than bedraggled. That's running to me."

CHAPTER 51
I run races with my husband and daughter
"More people would run if they took the time to take it easy first."

Suzie Oswald started running in 2005 at the age of 46. She and her husband were encouraged by their daughter to join the gym she works at. "We knew they had a program to train for the City to Surf in Sydney so we decided to have a go at it. We started out on the treadmill, getting very excited when we could manage 20 minutes without stopping. We still run because we enjoy the buzz we get from it. The only thing that has changed is the distance we run," Suzie says.

As residents of Port Macquarie, home to Ironman Australia, they find plenty of support for their running lifestyle. "There are lots of positive people around who love to run too and who are great for encouragement and helpful tips."

Suzie runs three times a week when she is preparing for a race, averaging 20km to 30km a week. She keeps track of her runs in a log book. She also works out at the gym and does boot camps. Suzie and her husband still train together.

"When we are injury-free it is a very important part of our weekly routine. Whether we are doing the same run we have done for ages or are trying to better our times, it still is a great buzz and a really good way to start the day. We like to run in the morning so if it means getting up a little earlier then we do it. I feel the heat and really don't enjoy running in the middle of the day or afternoon. I especially love the early winter mornings."

Suzie's family encourages her passion for running, especially her daughter who works at the gym and is studying to become a dietician. "She is fully aware of how much it means to me."

Not everyone is as understanding.

Some people think that her life these days revolves around the gym and running, she says. "I find the people who don't do much, or any, exercise in any form are the ones who think I am mad to want to run 21km."

Suzie has made new friends because of her running and enjoys the company of like-minded people. "Being fit is a lifestyle."

She loves the sensation that comes with a good run. "I feel on top of the world. It feels such an achievement to pull out a great run, especially when you look back and could only manage two minutes on the treadmill without collapsing in a heap. A great run inspires me to keep running and try more races."

She also has days when her session is a struggle. "It's amazing how hard you are on yourself but I am slowly learning that every run is different with different conditions. You have to just put them behind you and go on to the next, otherwise you would never run again. Most of the time it motivates me to try harder or try other training methods," Suzie says.

She only skips training sessions if she's injured. And then she doesn't feel guilty, especially if training would aggravate the injury. "I tore a quad muscle doing sprints which made me take it easy for a few weeks. I knew that if I didn't rush it, it would get better quicker."

Suzie definitely feels better after a run. She never lets her mood interfere with her running. "If it's a training day - regardless of my mood - I run. If my mood is crappy then by the time I have finished the run I am feeling a lot better."

Running has improved her quality of life. "It makes it easier to go to work. It wakes up the whole body and prepares you for the day ahead."

Running is important for her health and she is conscious of its health benefits. "I am 49 and find it a lot harder to keep the weight at an even level now than 10 years ago. But I don't exercise just for weight purposes.

"Overall I am very healthy with great cholesterol, bone density and blood pressure and I'd like to keep it that way."

Running is only part of her efforts to look after her health, along with the right nutrition. The same goes for her self-esteem and self-image. "It is an overall picture again: the running makes you feel great and you are happy with yourself so the self-esteem soars."

Suzie typically runs with others which she prefers. "I rarely run by myself. My husband is a great motivator and good to run with but I love to be in a group. I am presently doing a bootcamp-style of group fitness and it is great to be with a group as you can gauge your running with the fastest runner to extend yourself and take you out of your comfort zone. The social aspect of running is very important. You tend to bounce off other people's aims and achievements. It is great to be around like-minded people of all ages and abilities."

While she enters races, she says she is not competitive by nature. "I am happy to finish a race, rather than go hell for leather to make a great time and maybe not finish. I try to be consistent."

She hopes to keep running for a long time. "I haven't put a time limit on it. If I am fit and healthy and can run or go to the gym I will be doing it. I don't really think you can use age as an excuse. We have a guy of 74 in our local area and he is still competing in triathlons with great times. He's an inspiration to watch."

She has recommended running to others. "I tell them to start slow. I think so many more people would run if they took the time to take it easy first and not try to run too far. Then when you have confidence, choose a small fun run and give it a go. You just never know what you are capable of."

So far the 2007 Blackmores Bridge Run in Sydney was her best experience involving running. "My husband and I were training for it when I hurt my leg. He usually runs a lot faster than me and we usually meet up eventually at the finish line. This year he decided to run the whole way with me and we just took an easy pace and crossed the finish line together. It was a really great moment for us."

She cherishes the races in which their daughter ran as well. "It is a really great experience to all be at the finish line together."

The single-most important thing about running for Suzie is the ability to train and reach her goals. "The next one is hopefully to do a marathon. Running has made me so much more positive in everything I do."

CHAPTER 52
Running means fitness, friendship, enjoyment and challenge
"When I run I find myself in a space that I really like to be in."

Tara Baumann started running in 2001 when she was living and working in Canada. She joined a club because it had a program aimed at getting novice runners in shape to complete a 10km race. "Although I had run 5km now and again for fitness, I had never run beyond that distance. I decided that I really wanted to be able to run 10km, so I joined a running club that had a specific program for beginners."

Tara immediately took to the sport which was the reason for her to stick with it. "It was something that I really enjoyed. It made me feel good and I knew it aided a healthy lifestyle. The feeling that I got from running my first 10km race was great. I still get that feeling today when I finish a race where I know I have given it my best. What has changed for me in recent years is that I have become more goal-oriented with my running. I still hold the desire to run for enjoyment but at the same time challenge myself to achieve a pre-determined goal through a structured training program," she says.

Tara has also competed in a few triathlons but prefers running which is her main form of exercise. "These days I spend very little time in the water or on the bike. Although I know these two disciplines are great for cross-training, without a doubt my greatest passion is for running. When I run I find myself in a space that I really like to be in."

The frequency and intensity of her training varies, depending on the goal she is aiming for. She followed a training program for the 2007 Gold Coast marathon. "The program was structured specifically for me and my goals. It provided me with the structure and the discipline that I required. The program provided the guidance that I needed to train properly: when to run and when not to run, how far to run, how frequently to run and how fast to run for each session. It is important to train enough to get through a race but it is just as important not to overtrain."

She trained consistently for five months to prepare for that marathon, running six to seven times a week. "The intensity for each of these runs was different, ranging from long slow runs to shorter and faster runs, to very slow recovery runs," Tara says.

She keeps track of her training in a log book, recording her time out on the road and approximate kilometres covered on each run. For the 2007 marathon, her coach had her record her heart rate zones which she found aided her training significantly.

Running means many things to Tara including fitness, friendship, enjoyment and challenge. She generally has no trouble fitting it into her schedule because she makes it a priority. "Running has become part of my life. My partner is a keen runner also, which means we can spend time together while getting fit."

Their training has also turned into a way to hang out with friends. "We spend our Saturday mornings doing a long run with friends along the Brisbane River and then join them for breakfast afterward. In many ways running has become very social and a time to catch up with people."

Her training is challenging in the periods when her training volume for an event is at its highest. "It does become more difficult to fit everything in: early starts, fulltime work, some evening training sessions, social catch-ups with friends and family and the desire to have quality time at home make for a pretty full day."

People close to Tara are very supportive of her passion for running and she believes they completely understand what running means to her. "My partner shares my passion for running. Some of our friends have in fact been made through the running groups that we train with each week. My family always show an interest in my running, with my family cheering me on at the finish line of my last marathon. "Since then, my sister caught the bug and is kick-starting her training so she can participate in the Gold Coast 10km this year," Tara says.

Tara says the feeling that she has had a fantastic run can happen for many reasons. "For me a great run does not have to mean doing a great time in a race. A great run could be leaving the house on a beautiful sunny day and just enjoying the morning and observing the environment while running. It could be running 20km in the rain. It could be running through the trails of Mt Coot-tha or it could be slogging it out in a tough speed session. Sometimes a run can start difficult, with my legs feeling like lead, but by the end of it I am feeling great. Of course you can't go past the feeling of training hard and then achieving what you set out for on race day. But I know it has been a great run when I finish it and think, 'That was great'."

Tara usually doesn't skip training sessions, especially when she is on a specific program and is aiming for a goal. "There are occasions when other things in life take a priority. What I have learnt is that when a training session is skipped, don't try to make up for it by running further on your next training day, as this just leads to fatigue and a higher risk of injury."

After a layoff from training she finds it hard to get back into it initially. "When I stop running for a while, I do find it difficult to have that first run again and to get back into a consistent routine."

Tara likes to run with others as well as alone. "It is all about variety. For me, each group or run has its own purpose and benefit. I run with a mixed group of friends on the weekend because it is enjoyable and a good time to catch up. The social aspect helps me to complete a long run without even knowing I have covered the kilometres. During the week I train with organised groups of runners to do intervals and more demanding sessions that would be difficult to do on my own.

"Group training not only offers the social aspect to my running, but also the motivation to try harder. I also love to run alone and find time to do this each week as well," she says.

The social aspect of running is very important to Tara. "Running groups tend to attract fantastic, motivated and intelligent people who are fun to be around. I have met some great people through running."

CHAPTER 53
The social benefits of running are very important

"Running has improved my quality of life. I am happier and I have set goals to train for."

Toni Hackwill began running in June 2007 at the age of 44 after she and her husband had moved to Sydney five months earlier. They chose to join the Northside Running Group to follow a training program, thinking they'd kill two birds with one stone. "We needed to join a club to meet people plus I thought it would be good exercise to help lose a little bit of weight," says Toni who had only walked for exercise.

Since then Toni has consistently run three times a week. She has competed in a 5km race and the 9km Blackmores Bridge Run. Running across the Sydney Harbour Bridge was an experience she cherishes. Those races inspired her to increase her training frequency to four times a week because she plans to run a half marathon soon. While weight control is still a motivation for her running, she has found more important drivers. "I now run more for the social enjoyment and sense of accomplishment. Running means getting out in the fresh air, forgetting the stresses of life and feeling healthy," Toni says.

She has taken up Pilates, attending classes once a week, to underpin her run training through stretching and strengthening muscles. "I prefer running as I feel great afterwards."

Toni follows a training program and rarely skips workouts. And if she does skip one, she doesn't feel guilty. "There is no sense beating yourself up, I just admit that I missed a session and go onto the next one. I miss it greatly when I haven't been able to run but I find it easy to get back into it by doing a few shorter runs to start with," she says.

She keeps track her training in a spreadsheet, listing the time and distance she ran. She finds it easy to make running a part of her life. Training with a club is very motivating and Toni's husband is supportive since he also still trains with them. "We are both very passionate about running. My husband understands my love of running. But our families consider us to be obsessed."

Toni prefers training with others over solo runs. She has made new friends because of running and finds the social aspect of the sport important. "I prefer running in a group, especially being part of a running club where there is a mixed group. It is very important to chat to people before, during and after a run. I just like to have fun and keep it light-hearted."

In training she wants to push herself and tends to run at the front of the group. Even so she doesn't consider herself to be a competitive person. "I'm happy just to run in my own time."

Toni rewards herself for consistent training or reaching certain goals. "I usually treat myself to chocolate."

In the initial stages of her running Toni got injured. She had an Achilles tendon injury which stopped her running for three weeks. "It made more determined to get back to running and concentrate on preventing further injuries."

On a great run Toni feels happy and very energetic. A session during which she struggles leaves her feeling tired and quiet, she says. "A great run is when I feel happy whereas a crap run is when I feel down a little. It's definitely more mental than physical. A great run will boost my mood for days and I usually can't stop talking about it. I usually sleep off a run which hasn't been so good and it makes me train harder at the next session."

Toni finds it easier to go for a run when she is in a good mood. "I usually need a push when I am in a bad mood even though I know I will feel good afterwards. I feel better after a run than before a run. Running has improved my quality of life. I am happier and I have set goals to train for."

She considers running very important to her health and believes she is healthy because she runs. "I feel stronger, breathe easier and eat better. I am more aware of changes in my body and mental state."

Running is moderately important to her self-image. "It has been good to tone up and lose a little bit of weight."

She says that becoming a runner has changed her life. "I feel fitter and happier. I hope to be running when I am 75. For me, being a runner is definitely a lifestyle. Running is about feeling good with myself."

CHAPTER 54
This ultra-runner wants to run further

"They think I'm doing too much at my age or don't understand that even slow people can do races. But I have running friends."

Tina Fiegel started running in 1992 when she was in her early 40s. "I was inspired by Jane Fonda's book in which she talks about her quest to run a mile. I thought that I'd like to be able to run one kilometre," she says.

Tina has succeeded and then some. Her reasons to run today are similar to when she started but she has expanded her goals, and achievements, from that initial 1km. In 2006 the then 57-year-old ran 105.47 km (65.53 miles) in a 24-hour race. "It is still about fitness and a personal challenge but the distances are longer. It feels so good to stop. You feel really good and virtuous after a run."

She does other sports but running is near the top of her list. "Except for skiing, I prefer running. Running can be done everywhere, happens outdoors and often in scenic locations, is done to music and you get the very occasional runner's high. I run, therefore I am. Well not quite but it is a very important part of my life."

She runs between three and six times a week, with the sixth run done in water. Tina sets aside time for her running. "I make it fit. Mornings or evenings, it is a priority. I'm trying to build it up to five to six times a week consistently," she says.

She follows a training program because she wants to improve. She only skips training sessions if she's injured or if the weather is very bad. She feels guilty for skipping training. "I might modify the program, rather than skip it."

She certainly doesn't let a bad mood interfere with her running, and sometimes adds a session to improve it. "I usually run to a timetable. But when I'm angry I need a run more and might even do an extra one."

Tina keeps track of her runs in a log book to monitor her improvement, or lack thereof. It also allows her to understand what may have led to an injury of which she unfortunately has had a few. "I have had most running injuries and a few non-running ones. I couldn't wait to get going again and work on the recovery: one minute run, one minute walk..."

The people close to her are not supportive of her passion for running, she says. "They think I'm doing too much at my age or don't understand that even slow people can do races. But I have running friends."

People who also run do understand what running means to her – the ones who don't run do not comprehend, she says. Tina has made many new friends because of running. She says that she has probably also lost touch with some friends because of running. "I prefer to be around active people."

Tina has days when her running feels great and days when it is a struggle. The latter one leaves her feeling relieved that the session is finished, disappointed and often sore. "When it's a great run I feel elated, euphoric, happy, exhausted and sore."

The difference between feeling it has been a great run or a bad one depends on the time, pace or distance she has run. "It depends on whether I felt flat and sluggish or good doing it. It is more physical but it results in mental wellbeing." A great run will boost her mood for hours. A great race can lift her spirits for days.

She enters running races as a challenge and incentive to keep training. She says she is not a competitive person. "I'm happy for others to win. I'm competing against myself."

Tina enjoys running alone as well as with groups if she can. "I like running with other people, either women or men. But since I am very slow I usually run by myself. Being at a group training run or race helps, because there are people around. The social aspect of running is somewhat important but not essential."

Tina has recommended others to start running. "But they have to want to do it themselves. I don't try too hard to talk them into it."

Becoming a runner changed her life. She regards being a runner as a lifestyle. "I've always been active but now I'm more serious about this. I've gotten used to feeling pain and exhaustion and still keep going. It can interfere with your social life but the rewards are worth it. I try to keep it in balance."

She says that running has been a great improvement to her quality of life. "It keeps me fitter and more mobile - I'm 59 now and have arthritis - and it lifts my mood. I'd like to keep running until I drop dead. But I review this every five years or so. The longest I've done is a 24-hour track race. I would like to do a 48-hour race and the six-day race at Colac but I don't know whether my feet will let me."

She considers herself to be healthy because she runs. It is also important to her self-esteem and self-image, she says. "I'm an active person, a runner."

Finishing her first marathon is still her best experience involving the sport. "I experienced a real runner's high and had a big grin on my face, even though it hurt."

About the author

Margreet Dietz was born in 1970 in The Netherlands. After obtaining a Bachelor of Commerce, she began a career in marketing only to realise that what she really wanted to do was to write. She quit her job in 1995 and went back to school, moving to Brussels, Belgium, where she obtained a post-graduate degree in International and European Law. (Keep reading, it will soon make sense.) In 1996 she started working as a reporter at Bloomberg News in its Brussels office, followed by stints in Toronto, Canada, and subsequently Sydney, Australia. She left Bloomberg News in March 2004 to travel and compete in endurance sports events around the world including three Ironman triathlons. In 2006 she was hired as a copy-editor at The Australian Financial Review in Sydney, and began writing for endurance sports magazines. She followed her long-time partner Tim to the West Coast of Canada at the end of 2007, where she started researching and writing this book, her first. Margreet now lives with Tim and their dog Luka in Squamish, BC.

Made in the USA
Charleston, SC
17 February 2010